No. 4 in the Harnessing Health Information series

Series Editor
Michael Rigby

Harnessing Health Libraries

Bruce Madge

Radcliffe Medical Press

Radcliffe Medical Press
18 Marcham Road, Abingdon, Oxon OX14 1AA

British Library Cataloguing in Publication Data

A catalogue record for this book is available from the British Library.

ISBN 1 85775 408 5

Typeset by Joshua Associates Ltd, Oxford
Printed and bound by TJ International Ltd, Padstow, Cornwall

Contents

Preface

Harnessing Health Libraries

Libraries can be confusing places for the first-time user. Health libraries are no exception, and help to find exactly the article you are looking for can be vital, especially when meeting a tight deadline or trying to find evidence for a particular treatment. The rise of evidence-based healthcare has put a particular emphasis on finding the evidence, which may be in a specific journal article, and so a library is a place you need to know your way around.

As a health librarian for over 20 years in a variety of posts, from the National Health Service (NHS) to the British Library, I have had to track down a number of strange requests and I hope that this book reflects some of the knowledge I have gleaned. This book is designed to help the novice user to find what they are looking for in a library. It is designed as a 'how to' guide, admittedly written by a librarian but hopefully from a user perspective. It is not aiming to be a comprehensive treatise on medical librarianship in all its forms. Because of my current post, you may find a preponderance of information from the British Library, but I have tried to be as comprehensive and even-handed as possible. I would also like to take this opportunity to acknowledge the major part played in my early career by both John Mills, former Regional Librarian of South East Thames Regional Health Authority, and Shane Godbolt, Regional Librarian for North Thames Regional Health Authority – without their mentoring over the years this book would never have been written. I would also like to thank my mother, Delphine Madge, for her invaluable help with the index.

My aim is to help you, the reader, with the rudiments of finding health information before needing to seek detailed help from a librarian. I hope that I succeed in this endeavour.

Bruce Madge
January 2001

About the author

Bruce Madge has been Head of the Health Care Information Service at the British Library since 1995. He is head of the section that indexes the United Kingdom input into *Medline* for the US National Library of Medicine and which produces the popular *Allied and Complementary Medicine Database* (AMED).

He worked in NHS libraries in the South East for a number of years before being headhunted for the new post of Information Officer (Medical Informatics) at the British Medical Association (BMA). Here he built up their informatics collection, served on the BMA's IT Committee as well as representing the BMA on various external committees, and was instrumental in the BMA's work on the confidentiality of patient data.

From 1996 to 1998 he was Chair of the Health Libraries Group (HLG) of the Library Association, where he started the research panel to try to look at getting library research into practice. He also fostered the links between HLG and the British Medical Informatics Society, of which he is a member, with the aim of bringing health librarians and IT specialists closer together. In 2000 he became a National Councillor for the Library Association.

Since 1995 he has represented the British Library on the Library and Information Co-operation Council (LINC) Health Panel and is currently Chair-Elect of the International Co-operation Section of the Medical Library Association of the US. He also serves on the Committee of the Primary Health Care Specialist Group of the British Computer Society.

1 What is a health library?

Introduction to health libraries

Health is important to everyone and provides employment for a huge number of healthcare professionals. In the United Kingdom, the NHS is the country's largest employer. At some point during their training and work, all healthcare professionals need to access information which is to be found in a library, often with the help of a librarian. With the increased emphasis on 'evidence-based healthcare', a library has become an important source of evidence for treatment and increasingly librarians are learning how to critically appraise the literature that they retrieve.

A library, typically, may contain the following material:

- primary literature – i.e. books, journals and theses
- secondary literature – i.e. abstracting journals and databases containing details of articles published in the 'primary' literature
- grey literature – that material which does not have an International Standard Book or Serial Number (ISBN or ISSN) (*see below*), i.e. technical reports and reports from health authorities
- audio-visual media and multimedia.

But a library should not be seen purely as a static repository of materials especially with developments such as the Internet and the digital library, which will be discussed later.

Some history

Perhaps the most famous, and possibly the first, health library was the Great Library at Alexandria, where it is believed that the Hippocratic Corpus got its name because librarians had filed a series of medical texts together in the same place (perhaps the first instance of a medical classification scheme?). Some of the manuscripts were authored by the physician Hippocrates and so subsequently all the manuscripts, as they were kept together, were attributed to him.

Many of the first medical libraries were attached to universities. Christian monks in monasteries in Syria in the 10th and 11th centuries actually ran the first loans service between monasteries for the purpose of copying some of the surviving Greek medical texts. This helped to preserve works from Hippocrates and Galen, which in turn had a huge effect on the development of medicine in the West.

When the NHS was formed in 1948, libraries began to spring up in hospitals and then when Regional Health Authorities and District Health Authorities were formed in 1974, the King's Fund produced its seminal work on the role of a District Library Service.

The NHS reforms in the 1990s had an indirect impact on libraries. The main effect was that the funding streams changed as each trust became, in theory, self-funding. Most hospitals by this time had a library associated with a postgraduate medical centre, which catered mainly for doctors, and some had a nursing school with a library for students and on-site staff. By the end of the 1990s this had changed as training for nurses and other paramedical staff moved to higher education establishments. The quality of library provision for paramedical staff became variable in the move from the NHS to higher education and is only now settling down again.

A *Health Service Guideline HSG 97(47)* was produced in England because of concerns around the role and status of libraries within the NHS. The *HSG* acknowledged past problems including:

- the lack of a national policy for library and information services or clear national links to Research and Development, Education and Training, or Information Management and Technology strategies
- the complex funding arrangements whereby trust libraries receive funding from multiple sources, and funding streams for libraries which were difficult to identify
- uncertainty about capital funding for developing library and information services
- a legacy of libraries established to serve separate professional groups
- ambivalence about the range of staff groups which library services are funded to support, which could lead to inadequate services for nursing and other non-medical professional staff and community-based staff
- the transfer of nursing and midwifery education into higher education and the consequent closure or absorption of College of Health Libraries.

HSG 97(47) set out a number of key principles in relation to the development of library services.

- Access – NHS libraries should be multidisciplinary and meet the needs of all staff groups. NHS trusts and health authorities have a responsibility as good employers, and as providers and commissioners of high-quality evidence-based care, to ensure that all staff have access to the information needed to carry out their work effectively. Access policies should also consider the information needs of contractors, those undertaking career breaks and others.
- Resources – resources required to support an effective library service will vary according to local needs but will include a mix of professional and clerical library staff, and an appropriate range of books, journals, electronic information resources, computers and networks.
- Funding – the need for better co-ordination of funding streams for library services and greater clarity about the purposes and staff groups for which different funding streams are provided. The *HSG* proposed that access to library services should be free at the point of use, although charges may be levied for certain services.
- Region-wide co-ordination – there should be region-wide co-ordination of library services based on the key national principles of equity of access for all.

An information strategy context

Another major publication contributing to the future of libraries, but in a more indirect way, was *Information for Health*, which was described as 'A £1 billion investment to put information to work for NHS patients and staff'. It was decided that the NHS needed accurate and instantly accessible information which was vital for improving care for patients, the performance of the NHS and the health of the nation.

The aim of *Information for Health*, which applies to the NHS in England, is that it would help:

- doctors and nurses deliver better care by providing both up-to-the-minute details of the medical history of their patients and access to the latest medical research

- the NHS to ensure that it spends its £40 billion budget wisely and that all parts of the health service are working to the highest standards
- the public to be more involved in treatment decisions by giving them accurate information about their medical problems, and would provide reliable health information so they can stay fit and well.

Information for Health was designed to place greater emphasis on what is needed for treating patients rather than on administration, as in the past.

Over a period of time it is planned that the NHS will deliver:

- a lifelong Electronic Health Record for every person in the country
- instant access, 24 hours a day, in every hospital and GP's surgery to patient records and best clinical practice
- a National Electronic Library for Health to keep doctors and nurses up to date with the latest clinical research and best practice at the time they need it (more about this later)
- fast and convenient public access to information and care through on-line information services and telemedicine.

The vision was divided into two streams.

1 For the public

- New video and on-line technology is already being used to give patients and NHS medical staff access to specialists working at major centres of excellence. Telemedicine will increasingly eliminate the need for long, inconvenient and potentially dangerous journeys for patients.
- Linking GPs electronically to hospitals and chemists will reduce delays and anxiety in booking hospital appointments, receiving test results and checking on the availability of medicines.
- It will mean the end of frustrations and reduce the potential for mistakes in treating patients by making available the medical history of patients to their GPs and other authorised NHS professionals.
- Electronic Health Records and secure networks will improve confidence in the accuracy and confidentiality of medical records.
- NHS Direct is already successfully providing health advice over

the phone. The service will be extended to cover the whole country by the end of 2001. Together with new information services, an expanded NHS Direct will help provide a reliable source of NHS-approved advice on self-care and other health issues.

- Improved public information will be available on best medical practice through the new on-line services.

2 For NHS staff

NHS staff will share the benefits enjoyed by patients because much of the frustration felt through poor clinical records and co-ordination of services will be eliminated. But the new information technology will also bring other benefits to the NHS.

- It will give medical and nursing staff instant access, at their desks or at the bedside, to the most recent medical research and to treatment best practice.
- It will give better information to determine what works and what does not within the NHS. And it will enable the people making decisions over our £40 billion budget to ensure all sections of the NHS are working to the standards of the best.

The *Information for Health* strategy will also provide:

- a National Electronic Library for Health containing accurate information on the latest medical advances and accredited best practice guidance, with particular help on important topics
- early warning of regional variations or potential problems in clinical standards
- better information for public health doctors, planners and managers about priorities and effective approaches to improving healthcare and health.

Implementation of *Information for Health* was carried out through a series of consultations with NHS professions and public representatives, which discussed the principle of a national body to advise on patient confidentiality issues and its potential remit. The strategy proposed the connection of all computerised GP practices to NHSnet, so that GPs and hospitals could exchange information electronically about appointments and test results by the end of 1999, and to enable everybody in England to contact NHS Direct, the 24-hour nurse-led telephone advice line, by 2000. It also suggested the setting up of working groups of clinicians, managers and information specialists in every health authority area to plan the local implementation of the strategy and the setting up of 'beacon' sites to pioneer the development of Electronic Health Records. *Information for Health* also ensured that health authorities, trusts and primary care groups (PCGs) would receive the right support at national, regional and local level so that the NHS would successfully be able to implement the strategy and acquire the best services and systems, avoiding unnecessary duplication of effort.

However, even with these new directives from the NHS Executive, provision of library services to on-site nursing and other paramedical staff and to those in the community is still very patchy, but will hopefully be sorted out with the move towards electronic remote access.

The context of health libraries versus other libraries

There are many different types of library. Most people will have come across a local public library or a school library at some time in their lives. All libraries are arranged along similar lines, so by using a public library you will have some idea of the usual layout of a medical library. The major difference is usually the classification scheme used and the preponderance of books as opposed to journals. All public libraries use the Dewey Decimal classification scheme. This places most of the medical texts that a public library would stock, and which are usually aimed at the patient, in the 610 region, but more about that later. Marylebone Public Library in London is an example of a public library that collects medical texts – this is due to a scheme whereby each public library specialises in an area of the Dewey classification scheme.

Other types of library exist and some you will come across include academic and professional society libraries. Most schools and universities have libraries – medical schools are no exception and you will find that there is an induction course in library procedures within the first couple of weeks of starting a course. These libraries can use varying classification schemes, some of which are described below. Many universities have a medical school attached and so there is the possibility of having to deal with two different classification schemes depending on whether you are using the university library or the medical school library.

Then, of course, when you start in a professional post, the hospital will also have a library to which you will have access and which will allow you a variety of privileges, such as borrowing, ordering articles and searching databases. Most NHS libraries are now becoming multidisciplinary and so will allow all on-site health professionals to join; some are even offering services to patients as well. Some departments and wards will have a departmental collection of books and journals which cover the subjects they deal with all the time – this can be a source of keeping up to date with practice in your subject. It may also be useful to note that some hospitals have a library for patients, where a book trolley is trundled around the wards. These may be run by either the Red Cross or the local public library. It is not my intention here to deal with the subject of bibliotherapy, although there is a growing literature on the subject.

If you require more specialised services than those available in the professional library on-site, then a professional society library may be the answer, although it is perhaps inconvenient to travel to your professional headquarters every time you need to look at a book. Some libraries, e.g. the Wellcome Trust and the British Library, will allow users who can demonstrate a real need to get access to their collections.

Most public libraries will help you with interlibrary loans (*see* Chapter 6) if you cannot access a library in your own institution, but this procedure can be slower than using your own library and may be more expensive.

What health libraries contain and can help you with

Health libraries contain a wealth of information surrounding the field of healthcare practice and usually collect literature in the adjacent fields of social practice. In some cases, they will collect in more specialised areas, depending on any hospital specialities (e.g. the Institute of Cancer Research at the Royal Marsden Hospital will collect material mainly in the area of cancer research). Most will contain a collection of key reference texts such as dictionaries and encyclopaedias. Many will also have some sort of overnight loan collection where texts can be borrowed for a specified period and you are fined for not returning the book on time. It may be apocryphal, but there was a rumour that an American university library charged overdue fines by the second for their overnight loan collection!

Health libraries will also have access to bibliographic databases such as *Medline* on either CD-ROM or via the Internet and some are beginning to offer access to electronic versions of journals as full text on the Web.

Increasingly, public libraries are becoming especially interested in providing health information for patients and this will become progressively more important as a way of getting health information to patients and the public.

It should also be remembered that librarians in health libraries are trained as librarians first before specialising in health. Therefore they will have a knowledge of useful reference tools outside those specifically in the health field. They are also increasingly knowledgeable about the applications of information technology to information retrieval and the Internet. It is not unusual for libraries and librarians to develop skills in HTML (hypertext markup language) and JavaScript to write web pages about their collections. Examples are the South Thames Library page at http://www.lib.surrey.ac.uk/STHAMES/STLIS/stlis.htm, which also provides information about the postgraduate dean and training programmes for medical staff, and Project Connect, which does the same for North Thames at http://www.nthames-health.tpmde.ac.uk/ntrl/welcome.htm

The role of libraries in the evidence-based age

With the advent of 'evidence-based medicine' (EBM), first in Canada at McMaster University and then throughout the UK, the profile of librarians has been raised. This is due to their role in the literature-searching part of the evidence-based movement. Because of the necessity of tracking down the literature on particular therapeutic interventions and finding the 'gold standard' – the randomised controlled trial – librarians had a major role to play and also extended their services into the whole arena of critical appraisal of the results of the literature search. The major resource for EBM and the wider area of evidence-based healthcare is the *Cochrane Library* produced from the work of the Cochrane Collaboration and used to support its continuing work. The *Cochrane Library* consists of a number of databases which can be cross-searched; these include:

- the *Cochrane Database of Systematic Reviews* (*CDSR*)
- the *Database of Abstracts of Reviews of Effectiveness* (*DARE*)
- the *Cochrane Controlled Trials Register* (*CCTR*).

It also incorporates the *Cochrane Review Methodology* database (which is a bibliography of articles on methods or research synthesis), a handbook on critical appraisal, a glossary of terms and a list of sources of evidence on the Internet called *Netting the Evidence* (*see below*). The CD-ROM and web version (at http://www.update-software.com) is provided by Update software. The *DARE* database is available free on-line via the NHS Centre for Reviews and Dissemination (NHS CRD) at the University of York (http://nhscrd.york.ac.uk/welcome.html).

Also produced by the NHS, using Update software and of use in EBM, is the *National Research Register* (*NRR*) which lists current research being performed in the NHS for NHS staff needing to know the results of research or for those involved in commissioning research. The records are indexed using the National Library of Medicine's Medical Subject Headings (*MeSH* – *see below*) terms and include, among other information, details of research titles, methodology and outcome measures. In addition, the *NRR* contains the *MRC Trials Directory*, reviews in progress at the NHS CRD and ongoing research at the Centre for Health Economics at York. It is available on a CD-ROM, via the Internet and most NHS libraries will have access to the database.

Also of use in EBM and found in many NHS libraries is *Best Evidence*, the electronic marriage of *ACP Journal Club* and *Evidence-Based Medicine*. The *ACP Journal Club on Disk*, which consisted of the cumulated contents of *Journal Club* since its beginning in 1991, was launched in July 1995. *Evidence-Based Medicine* was added in July 1996 and the combined product was named *Best Evidence* from the January 1997 issue.

Best Evidence allows you to access precise summaries of the best current studies of diagnosis, cause, course and management of a broad range of clinical disorders. All the studies from 1991 have been thoroughly reviewed by authors and commentators, eliminating all outdated studies and upgrading the remaining reports to 1996 reporting standards. Over 90% of the 1991 studies are still of current relevance, reflecting the rigorous standards all studies must meet when first selected. The database can be searched by simple full-text searching or through index terms. The electronic version also contains the cumulative glossary of terms that was begun in 1996 in *Evidence-Based Medicine. Best Evidence* is available as a yearly CD-ROM on subscription from the American College of Physicians, the Canadian Medical Association and the BMJ Publishing Group. *Best Evidence* is also part of *Evidence-Based Medicine Reviews* from OVID Technologies.

As EBM grows in importance we have seen a number of 'evidence-based' journal titles ranging from medicine to nursing and specific topics such as child health and cardiology. A new publication which probably points to the direction in which EBM publications will go is *Clinical Evidence*, produced by BMJ Publishing Group and designed to sit in a healthcare professional's pocket alongside the *British National Formulary* and to be updated regularly.

There is also a very useful website which can keep you up to date with the latest developments in evidence-based healthcare. It is hosted by the School of Health and Related Research at Sheffield (ScHARR) and is maintained by the Information Service – it is called *Netting the Evidence: A ScHARR Introduction to Evidence Based Practice on the Internet* (http://www.shef.ac.uk/~scharr/ir/netting/net.html) and is also available as part of the *Cochrane Library*.

Further reading

Burns F (1998) *Information for Health: an information strategy for the modern NHS 1998–2005*. NHS Executive.

Department of Health (1997) *Library and Information Services, HSG (97) 47*. Department of Health, London.

King Edward's Hospital Fund for London King's Fund Centre (1985) *Providing a District Library Service: proposals arising from a series of workshops held in 1983 about the contribution library services can make to the provision of information in the NHS*. King Edward's Hospital Fund for London King's Fund Centre, London.

Roberts R (1999) *Information for Evidence-based Care. Harnessing Health Information Series No.1* Radcliffe Medical Press, Oxford.

2 Understanding the library

Library arrangement schemes

The most important part of a healthcare library will be the periodicals collection. This is due to the nature of medical publishing and knowledge – most important new work is disseminated quickly in periodicals, whereas a textbook may take two years to be published and so cannot contain current research. Most libraries will have a current listing of their periodical holdings and some will have lists of other libraries to which they have access. Most will be in alphabetical order by title, but a word of warning, some libraries (including the British Library) will list journals by professional bodies under that body's name first, i.e. instead of *Journal of the Royal Society of Medicine*, the list will say *Royal Society of Medicine, Journal*. This is often misleading and can lead users to believe that a common journal is not stocked in the library.

Journals are usually arranged on shelves alphabetically, although some libraries still place journals in classified order on the shelves. This can make them more difficult to find and, in an era of rising database usage to find references, is now probably unnecessary. It is also difficult to justify the practice when topics are increasingly being found in journals that are not necessarily on the subject, i.e. a lot of HIV/AIDS literature is found in journals such as the *BMJ* and the *Lancet*.

Some libraries may shelve the most important journals in a separate section or place the current issues on a separate rack. Current issues are then bound and placed on the shelves, the coverage and back runs being available on the open shelves. This varies from one library to another; for instance the British Library and the BMA Library keep only the last ten years of journals available on the open shelves and collections before that time are placed in basement storage.

Book catalogues and classification schemes

Most proper libraries are arranged in some sort of classification order. However, departmental libraries, especially those in the NHS, tend historically to be unclassified and are usually arranged by title or date. Where librarians have been involved in organising departmental collections, there is usually some sort of listing or basic classification scheme. The major classification schemes are detailed below.

All health libraries will have a catalogue. These are compiled using standard rules which make them consistent, and therefore searching a catalogue in one library will be much the same as searching a catalogue in the next library you come to. These rules are called the *Anglo–American Cataloguing Rules* (*AACR2*).

The catalogue could either be a card catalogue on the standard 5″ × 3″ cards, a book-form catalogue, a microfiche version or on computer, such as an OPAC (Online Public Access Catalogue). Increasingly, OPACs are appearing on the Internet so that potential users can identify what materials a library stocks before making a trip to consult the collection. Card catalogues tend to be disappearing due to space limitations in libraries; microfiche catalogues are also on the decline in the era of CD-ROM – for instance *SCICAT*, which is the catalogue of the British Library's Science Collection, was on microfiche until 1997 when it was superseded by a CD-ROM version and this has now been withdrawn in favour of Internet access.

One system which you may still see is a Kardex system for recording serial issue receipts. This is a system of shallow trays with cards which have the name of the journal written on the bottom edge. By lifting up the previous card you can see a grid which shows which, along with other information, issues have been received by the library. This system is gradually being replaced by computerised systems, but this whole process seemed to present a problem for computer programmers as successful systems which were quicker to use were very slow to appear and may still actually be slower than the well-tried Kardex system.

You will find that where card catalogues still exist, there are a number of sequences – an author sequence arranged by author surname (typically), a subject heading sequence which will probably be based on the classification scheme used, a dictionary catalogue where authors, subjects and certain other entries are arranged in one alphabetical sequence, and a classified catalogue arranged in the same subject order as the classification scheme used by the library.

The catalogue entry will, at a minimum, show author, title, publisher, date and shelf mark – traditionally in the top right-hand corner of the card. Some will go into greater detail and include page numbers, illustrations, size and subject heading. An example of a complete catalogue entry can be seen by looking at the reverse of the title page of a book published in America which shows a typical Library of Congress entry.

Both card catalogues and OPACs will allow searching by author, title and subject. Some OPACs will also allow searching by ISBN and ISSN number (*see below*) or by publisher or the keywords in a title.

Two methods of arrangement in alphabetical order may become apparent in catalogues, word by word or letter by letter – the first being the more popular.

Word by word	*Letter by letter*
New, John	New, John
New Forest	Newark
New Sydenham Society	New Forest
Newark	Newspapers
Newspapers	New Sydenham Society

Proper names beginning with M, Mac, Mc, St are arranged as if spelt Mac or Saint, and personal and proper names which contain apostrophes are treated as one word. Other characters in German or Scandinavian are treated as diphthongs.

Computer catalogues are basically databases with searching features available on selected fields. You are usually presented with a login feature where you enter a user name and password. In a large library you may have a choice of catalogues to search or these may be amalgamated into one large database. For instance, the British Library OPAC allows you to select between the Humanities catalogues (pre- and post-1975) and the Science and Technology catalogues. Of course, this throws up difficulties in knowing where a book would be situated, especially in the areas of the social sciences. However, there is cross-catalogue searching and the new catalogue which will be available soon will remove this obstacle.

Searches can be made by typing in author names, words in the title, publisher or ISBN/ISSN; further refinements can then be made if the retrieval numbers are too large. Some OPACs allow Boolean searching and truncation (*see* Chapter 4). Most systems will allow browsing through the list of authors or subjects.

OPACs on the Internet

There are increasing numbers of OPACs now available on the Internet. Most can be found through the NISS (National Information Services and Systems) website (http://www.niss.ac.uk). NISS also offers links to useful reference works, job details and other information – it is a useful starting place to look for OPACs. Some OPACs require a password to access them, but these are usually supplied on the first page of the OPAC and allow searching for reference purposes. A facility like this can be extremely useful for locating materials which are available locally or within reasonable travelling distance. However, a phone call to the library is always advisable to check on both the access rules and the availability of the item. Most OPACs offer the same breadth of searching, so once you have searched one, you can probably handle most of them.

A good example of a freely available OPAC is the British Library's own OPAC97. This can be found at www.bl.uk/opac97 and lists material held by both the London Reading Rooms reference collections and the Document Supply Centre at Boston Spa. You can select which collection you wish to search (left side London materials, right side Document Supply materials) and then search on author, title, publisher, ISBN/ISSN, etc. Truncation is a colon, i.e. 'heal:' will give you health, healthy and healthier as well as healing or healer. The retrieved items come up as a brief list and you can then link to a more detailed record which gives you a shelf mark and holding records.

If you are based in London and are looking for journals, the *London University Union List of Serials* is a good starting place. This is still a text-based telnet application (telnet://uls.qmw.ac.uk) but a series of search screens allows you to look for specific titles and their locations in London.

For readers outside the UK there are a number of excellent OPACs, the best possibly being the *Locator Plus* offered by the National Library of Medicine (NLM) (http://www.nlm.nih.gov/locatorplus/locatorplus.html). This replaced the *CATLINE*, *AVLINE* and *SERLINE* databases which had been offered by the NLM since the mid-1960s. *Locator Plus* allows searching of the complete collections of the NLM, which includes audio-visual (AV) materials as well as book and journals.

Other worldwide OPACs can be accessed through *Webcat* (http://

www.lights.com/webcats), which allows geographical searching and appears to be fairly comprehensive.

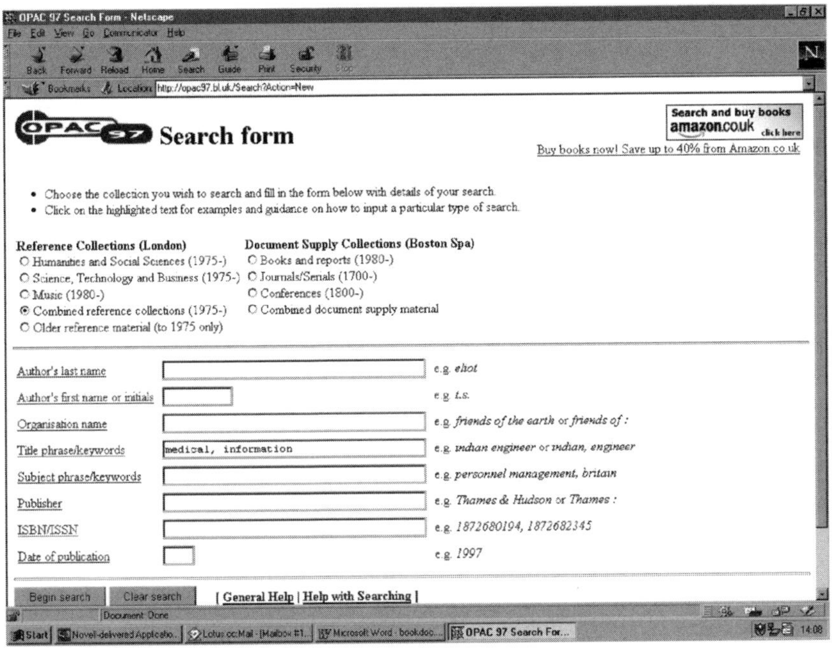

Figure 2.1 The British Library's OPAC

British National Bibliography (*BNB*)

The on-line source of the printed *British National Bibliography* contains bibliographic records for books and first issues of serial titles in the UK and Republic of Ireland. The current file, updated weekly, also holds details of forthcoming books and serial titles under the Cataloguing-in-Publications programme. Records are in UKMARC format, catalogued to AACR2 standard, with full subject indexing. The database is available as a print version, a CD-ROM and on-line via the British Library's own service and EINS (European Information Network Services – *see below*).

Whitakers Books in Print

The on-line equivalent of *British Books in Print*, holding records of British books and English-language books published overseas but available from a UK distributor. The file is updated monthly, contains current information on price and availability, and permits searches for in-print, out-of-print and forthcoming titles. It is available from 1956 onwards either on-line for a fee or as a CD-ROM by subscription.

Subject headings

Subject headings in a catalogue are usually based on an accepted thesaurus of medical terms. The most comprehensive is *Medical Subject Headings* (*MeSH*) produced and updated annually by the NLM. Originally *MeSH* was produced to subject index the printed *Index Medicus* and then the *Medline* database. As an American product, there are some modifications needed to the spelling (i.e. paediatrics instead of pediatrics) and some terms vary between the US and UK, i.e. acetaminophen and paracetamol. It includes cross-references to synonyms and alternative terms and the whole is based on tree structures of terms which will be illustrated in Chapter 4. *MeSH* is now available for searching on the Web through the NLM site (http://www.nlm.nih.gov/mesh/meshhome.html) and this makes it far more flexible as a retrieval tool.

A recent development at the NLM is the *Unified Medical Language System* (*UMLS*) which is attempting to map coding and subject heading schemes together to allow for better searching of terms in both the literature and the medical record. For instance, by searching for 'heart attack' the *UMLS* system will map to the preferred term 'myocardial infarction' and then give the user a list of terms which include the *International Classification of Diseases 9th and 10th edition* codes and the *Read Codes* used by GPs. Work is continuing on this project which will be essential for the linking of medical knowledge to the electronic patient record.

ISBNs and ISSNs

ISBN and ISSN are seen as some sort of mystical acronyms talked about by librarians. The International Standard Book Number (ISBN) and the International Standard Serial Number (ISSN) are unique numbers assigned to a book or journal title by its publisher. By knowing the ISBN or ISSN of a publication, a book or journal can easily be tracked on an OPAC when author or title details are sketchy. ISBNs are assigned to publishers in blocks, so the first few numerals are unique to each publisher and the last number is a check digit to make sure that the number is correct. ISSNs are supplied in the UK by the British Library ISSN centre – each new journal is assigned a unique number to identify it.

Classification schemes

Classification schemes may be designed as general schemes to cover the whole of knowledge or as special subject classification schemes. As the stock in a health library has to cover the whole of medical knowledge, classification schemes have grown up just to cover the health area. Some of these are based on classifications of disease.

Most health libraries now use one of these specialised schemes, although some still use a general scheme or their own 'home-grown' classification scheme (e.g. the British Library Science, Technology and Business collection). Home-grown classifications and general classification schemes in health libraries are beginning to die out in favour of more specific health-related classifications such as the NLM scheme.

The descriptions below are brief and health-specific. Each library will be able to supply more details about its own scheme to interested readers.

Dewey Decimal classification

Dewey is a general scheme covering the whole of human knowledge but very much based on 'Victorian values', so more space is given to religion and philosophy than the sciences. As mentioned above, public libraries favour the Dewey system and that is the classification with which most people will be familiar. There are ten main classes numbered 0 to 9. Further subdivisions are made by adding numbers to the right of the main number and by using decimal numbers; a point is added after the third number. This allows indefinite expansion but it can separate literature dealing with various aspects of a system, organ or region.

6	Useful arts			
61		Medicine		
611			Anatomy	
611.1				Cardiovascular system
612			Physiology	
612.1				Cardiovascular system
616			Internal and clinical medicine	
616.1				Cardiovascular system
616.12				Heart disease

Other tables allow an indication of language and time, etc.

Universal Decimal Classification (UDC)

UDC is an expansion of Dewey and allows for more detailed classification of topics with the consequent problem that numbers can become very long and unwieldy. It is favoured by some university libraries.

Library of Congress scheme

This is a general scheme more popular in university libraries than in health libraries. It uses a mixed notation, alphabetical and numerical. The major fields are alphabetical with a second letter to indicate subdivisions. Further subdivisions are by number. Class Q covers science, which includes laboratory science and pre-clinical subjects, while R is the shelf mark for medicine. It is an excellent scheme for general libraries but tends to separate information on regions of the body, organs and systems.

Bliss classification

This is another very detailed general scheme but used by some health libraries. It is an alphabetical and faceted scheme and has recently been looked at again with the rise of the topic of knowledge management. Class H covers anthropology, human biology and health sciences. It uses a preferred citation order: 1 – Person; 2 – Part, organ or system; 3 – Process; 4 – Action; 5 – Agent; although allowance is made for alternative citation orders.

HWE	Respiratory system				
HWF		Pharynx			
HWFT			Tonsils		
HWFT GL				Surgery	
HWFT GNG					Tonsillectomy

National Library of Medicine classification scheme

The NLM scheme is now the most used scheme in health libraries, for which it was purposely designed. It is a development of the Library of Congress scheme and is alphabetical and numerical in nature. Pre-clinical sciences are classified under QS–QZ and the clinical sciences are under the letter W, both of which were undeveloped in the original Library of Congress scheme.

WB Practice of medicine
WG Cardiovascular system
WG 200 Heart, general works
WG 201 Anatomy, histology, embryology
WG 202 Physiology, mechanisms of heartbeat
WG 205 Cardiac emergencies

Many NHS libraries use the system and have made regional modifications to include new topics, as revision of the scheme tends to be slow. Many libraries do not use the nursing section, except for general books on the nursing profession, preferring to file the nursing books with the topic that they are about – so paediatric nursing will be filed with the paediatrics books. QS (Anatomy, histology and embryology) and QT (Physiology) are used for general books on the subject, while books about specific systems are placed with the system as in the example (WG 201). Books outside of these fields are classified using the Library of Congress scheme.

Barnard classification

The Barnard scheme was devised by Cyril Barnard, the late librarian of the London School of Hygiene and Tropical Medicine, in 1936. It was revived in 1955, and an attempt to revise it in the 1970s and 1980s met with no success. It is still used at the London School of Hygiene and Tropical Medicine with local amendments, at the Royal College of Obstetricians and Gynaecologists, and at one point was the classification scheme used by the World Health Organisation (WHO). However, most other health and medical libraries have dropped it in favour of the NLM classification scheme. It is a specific classification, all aspects of one topic being in one place, and it is alphabetical.

O Cardiology
OA Blood pressure
OB Hypertension
OOJ Heart failure
OOJ.RRV Catheterisation of the heart

'.RRV' is the specific class mark for intubation or catheterisation.

Further reading

Morton LT, Wright DJ (1990) *How to Use a Medical Library* (7e). Clive Bingley, London.

3 Key special collections in health

Introduction

The Directory of Medical and Health Care Libraries in the United Kingdom and the Republic of Ireland, published by the Library Association and now in its 8th edition, and the *Guide to Libraries and Information Sources in Medicine and Health Care*, edited by Peter Dale, 2nd edition published by the British Library, provide details of most of the healthcare libraries in the UK. Similar lists exist for libraries in North America and the rest of the world.

The following are some of the major health collections which can be accessed in the UK, and one of the major international collections at the NLM in Washington DC.

The British Library, 96 Euston Road, London NW1 2DB. Tel: 020 7412 7288; http://www.bl.uk

The British Library is the national library of the UK and as such is a general library situated on three sites. The British Library is a legal deposit library and therefore receives all material published in the UK – it does not, as popular rumour has it, have every book ever published.

The London reading rooms are at St Pancras and Colindale (the Newspaper Library), and the Document Supply Centre (DSC) is in Boston Spa in Yorkshire. The collections are listed on OPAC97 (*see* page 14) for outside consultation and the internal OPAC is available for consultation in the entrance hall at St Pancras. Although the library is a general collection and not promoted specifically as a health library, there is a raft of health and medically related material in the collections and their general nature allows access to subject areas which may be of interest to healthcare practitioners, such as social services and community care. The periodicals held are listed on the website as well as printed in the *Current Serials in the British Library* publication which is issued annually. Hand lists of journals are also available for readers in the reading rooms.

Access to the collections is by reader's pass which can be obtained by filling in an application form available from the readers' admission office in the front hall at St Pancras. Passes range from one month to five years and will allow users access to all the collections held in the British Library at St Pancras for reference purposes only. The huge Document Supply Collections at Boston Spa may also be accessed from St Pancras with a 24-hour turnaround period. The Newspaper Library at Colindale operates on a similar system.

The DSC at Boston Spa does possess a reading room but a phone call is required to ascertain whether there is room available (tel: 01937 546000). From this reading room one can access the vast collections of the British Library DSC which provides a back-up service for most of the libraries in the UK and many around the world. For borrowing purposes it is recommended that a user consults their local library first and carries out an interlibrary loan (*see* Chapter 6).

The Health Care Information Service of the British Library (tel: 020 7412 7489) provides a quick enquiry service on health-related issues and the collections of the British Library available for consultation. There is also a service for more in-depth enquiries which is fee-based and aimed at small to medium companies.

The British Medical Association, BMA House, Tavistock Square, London WC1H 9JP. Tel: 020 7383 6625; http://www.bma.org.uk

The BMA Library is one of the three largest medical libraries in London (the British Library and the Royal Society of Medicine (RSM) Library being the other two). It is a membership library primarily aimed at members of the Association but open to other healthcare professionals on a day-ticket basis for a fee. The collection is chiefly clinical but the coverage is in great depth and there is an excellent AV collection. The BMA Library also provides document supply and loans to both personal members and over 600 institutional members, the vast majority of which are NHS libraries. A good way therefore to access the BMA collection is via a local NHS library. The BMA also runs a successful *Medline* search service for BMA personal members.

The Royal Society of Medicine, 1 Wimpole Street, London W1M 8AE. Tel: 020 7290 2940; http://www.rsm.org.uk

The RSM Library is the other major collection in London and covers a wider range of material than the BMA, including many statistical works and research-level material. It is also a membership library but has a day-ticket system for a fee. If regular use of the collection is foreseen then becoming a fellow of the RSM may be worth considering.

The Wellcome Trust, 183 Euston Road, London NW1 2BE. Tel: 020 7611 8582; http://www.wellcome.ac.uk

The Wellcome Trust has two main collections – the Library of the Institute for the History of Medicine and the Library and Information Service. The former is based on the private collections of Henry Wellcome (1853–1936), the pharmaceutical chemist. As such it has an unsurpassed collection of historical materials from around the world. The Wellcome also has a publicly accessible Information Service which contains many basic texts and is aimed firmly at supporting the public understanding of science. Both libraries are open to the general public for consultation purposes. The institute also produces the monthly *Current Work in the History of Medicine* which lists all the major articles and new books on the subject. Several editions of their catalogue were printed but it is now available on the Web.

The King's Fund, 11–13 Cavendish Square, London W1M 0AN. Tel: 020 7307 2568; http://www.kingsfund.org.uk/

The King's Fund library is the premier source for information on healthcare management. Compared to the other libraries, it is a recent collection but very comprehensive. It is open to healthcare professionals and to the public.

The Royal Colleges

Most of the Royal Colleges possess a library which is for use by their members, the exceptions being the Royal College of General Practitioners and the Royal College of Psychiatrists which have closed their libraries in favour of information centres. Psychiatry is well covered by the Institute of Psychiatry, a University of London institute attached to the Maudsley Hospital in Denmark Hill, South London. Other Royal Colleges exist in Scotland (the Royal Colleges of Physicians and of Surgeons in Glasgow and Edinburgh) and in Ireland (especially the Royal College of Surgeons of Ireland in Dublin). All have excellent historical collections but also provide up-to-date information services for their members. For nursing material, the Royal College of Nursing houses a major collection of both current and historical material. Another significant collection of nursing literature is the Nightingale Collection at St Thomas' Hospital.

Other professional associations

The libraries of both the Chartered Society of Physiotherapy (CSP) and the College of Occupational Therapists (COT) deserve mention as they serve their respective constituencies as major collections.

The CSP library (http://www.csp.org.uk) is situated at 14 Bedford Row, London WC1R 4ED (tel: 020 7306 6666, also the Information Resource Centre 020 7306 6605/4), while COT (http://www.cot.co.uk) is at 106–114 Borough High Street, Southwark, London SE1 1LB (tel: 020 7450 2316 (direct), 020 7357 6480 (switchboard); fax: 020 7450 2364/2299).

Both have extensive collections in their respective areas and hold a number of electronic resources.

Academic institutions

The first chair of medicine in Britain was established at Aberdeen University in 1495. At present many of the older universities and some of the 'new' universities offer medical and healthcare professional teaching and therefore support a health library. In recent years the University of London has merged medical schools under 'umbrella' universities, so that Imperial College for instance now has five medical school libraries under its umbrella. The University of London has also created a number of institutes over the years that have excellent libraries and are available to University of London students. These include the Institute of Neurology, Institute of Ophthalmology, Institute of Child Health, etc.

Research institutions

The National Institute of Medical Research at Mill Hill, which is one of the Medical Research Council's institutions, has a major library. It has an outstanding collection of research material available to its own staff and to other libraries via interlibrary loan. Other institutions with major libraries include the Central Public Health Laboratory at Colindale and the Imperial Cancer Research Fund at Lincoln's Inn Fields.

Further afield

While many of these major libraries are situated in London, there are other notable collections in health institutions around the country and many have counterparts around the world. Although it is in the US, the National Library of Medicine (NLM) deserves a place in any book on health libraries.

The National Library of Medicine, 8600 Rockville Pike, Bethesda, MD 20894; http://www.nlm.nih.gov

The NLM, on the campus of the National Institutes of Health (NIH) in Bethesda, Maryland, is the world's largest medical library. The library collects materials in all areas of biomedicine and healthcare, as well as works on biomedical aspects of technology, the humanities, and the physical, life, and social sciences. The collections stand at 5.8 million items – books, journals, technical reports, manuscripts, microfilms, photographs and images; there is also one of the world's finest medical history collections of old and rare medical works. The library's collection may be consulted in the reading room or requested on interlibrary loan in the US or through the network of Medlars Centre around the world. NLM is a national resource for all US health science libraries through the National Network of Libraries of Medicine.

Research and development in the fields of librarianship and informatics is carried out by the Lister Hill National Center for

Biomedical Communications (LHNCBC) and the National Center for Biotechnology Information (NCBI). The LHNCBC explores the uses of computer, communication and AV technologies to improve the organisation, dissemination and utilisation of biomedical information. The Lister Hill Center has conducted a number of valuable experiments using NASA satellites, microwave and cable television, and computer-assisted instruction. Currently the centre is applying modern communications technologies to healthcare-related projects involving, for example, telemedicine, testbed networks, virtual reality and other major projects.

The NCBI is developing information services for biotechnology – the task of storing and making accessible the staggering amounts of data about the human genome resulting from genetic research at the NIH and laboratories around the nation. NCBI also distributes GenBank, a collection of all known DNA sequences, and maintains the Human Gene Map on the World Wide Web at (http://www.ncbi.nlm.nih.gov/genemap).

The Toxicology and Environmental Health Program (TEHIP), established in 1967, is charged with setting up computer databases from the literature and from files of governmental and non-governmental organisations.

The NLM also organises tours of the building on Mondays through to Fridays.

4 Finding published materials

Introduction

In the previous chapter we have discussed how to find book material and where the major collections are housed. This chapter aims to look at the major source of information to support healthcare, which is mainly found in the journal literature.

The journal literature

A journal or serial or periodical publication may be defined as a publication issued in successive parts which is planned to continue indefinitely. Works such as *Annual Reviews* and the *Yearbook* series are periodicals, whereas conference proceedings and technical reports are not considered as such. A health library will contain many periodicals as they are the primary means of reporting research and are published on a very rapid turnaround – weekly, monthly or quarterly. A good health library can be judged on the number of journals that it holds as opposed to textbooks or reference works. Much of the library budget will go on journals and various methods for storing them.

It is difficult to ascertain the number of health-related journals today, although Wyatt (1991) estimated about 32 000 compared with just 1654 in 1912. The health literature has exploded exponentially and this has led to the problem of 'information overload' in the health profession. However, recent estimates put the number of journals at between 14 000 and 15 000 as journals not only are born but also die.

As mentioned in Chapter 1, there are two types of periodical literature – primary literature, with journals such as the *Lancet*, the *BMJ*, etc., and secondary literature which includes abstracting journals and indexes such as *Index Medicus*. Some authors also refer to tertiary journals which they classify as those journals containing reviews, such as the *Annual Review of Biochemistry*.

Search tools

To access this vast wealth of health information has become easier over the past 30 years with the advent of computer searching. To track the literature before this time, you will need to turn to the printed abstracting and indexing journals, of which some of the major ones are listed here.

Most of the printed indexes and abstracts are now available electronically but to search the literature before the 1960s you will need to use the printed versions of these electronic databases. Actually tracking down printed indexes can be hard work as more and more libraries discard print in favour of electronic access.

Surgeon General's Catalogue

The US produces the most important indexes of medical literature. The first of these was the *Index-catalogue of the Surgeon General's Office* which was conceived by John Shaw Billings, a distinguished American librarian. He produced a specimen catalogue in 1876 which was well received and so he proceeded with the *Index-catalogue*. The first volume appeared in 1880 and publication continued annually with each volume covering a different letter of the alphabet. When the alphabet was completed a new series was begun, again working through the literature and picking up new material which had been received by the library. Publication ceased in the middle of the fourth series owing to its inability to cope with the huge growth in the medical literature. Also due to the alphabetical nature of the publication, some material might wait 20 years before getting on to the list.

The volumes that are available are:

- 1st Series: Vol. 1–16 1880–95
- 2nd Series: Vol. 1–21 1896–1916
- 3rd Series: Vol. 1–10 1918–32
- 4th Series: Vol. 1–11 (A–Mn) 1936–55

A fifth series containing selected books appeared in three volumess 1959–61. Various supplementary catalogues have been released since and the *NLM Current Catalogue* is the latest version of this vast undertaking. Although it only lists the holdings of the Surgeon General's Library (later the National Library of Medicine), people consider it to be a complete list of the medical literature from the advent of printing to the middle of the 20th century. It should be remembered, however, that many books did not appear until years after they were printed, or were included when the library bought them; also Billings was fairly selective as to which periodical literature should be included.

In 1966 the NLM brought out its *NLM Current Catalogue*, which appeared twice a month with quarterly and annual cumulations. However, in 1993 this publication ceased and all the catalogues became electronically searchable (*see* Chapter 2 about *Locator Plus*).

Index Medicus

Index Medicus has had a chequered career, being produced in various editions by the NLM and the American Medical Association at various times. It has also changed its name to *Quarterly Cumulative Index Medicus* and to *Current List of Medical Literature* during its lifetime to satisfy the demand for up-to-date listings of the periodical literature. In January 1960 the *Current List* was replaced by *Index Medicus*, which was published monthly and cumulated annually. Currently *Index Medicus* is produced by the NLM, covers about 4000 titles and cumulates annually into 14 volumes which are classified by author and subject using the *MeSH* subject headings. For some years in the 1980s and 1990s there was an *Abridged Index Medicus* which contained the 120 most popular medical journals, but this has since ceased publication. *Index Medicus* is perhaps best known as the printed version of the *Medline* database.

The NLM also produces a series of *Current Bibliographies in Medicine* which cover a number of up-to-the-minute topics (e.g. telemedicine). These are available freely from the Web via the NLM home page (http://www.nlm.nih.gov).

Current Contents

Current Contents is produced by the Institute for Scientific Information (ISI) and is a weekly current awareness tool consisting of reproductions of the contents pages of about 7000 journals and some books. The three of most interest in the health field are *Current Contents: Life Sciences* (1379 titles), *Current Contents: Clinical Medicine* (1083 titles) and *Current Contents: Social and Behavioral Sciences* (1596 titles). There is some overlap between the titles. Each issue contains a selective list of book series, reviews and proceedings as well as list of journals, a subject index and the addresses of the first author of each article appearing. An updated list of the journals covered is produced twice a year.

Science Citation Index

Also produced by ISI, *Science Citation Index* and *Social Science Citation Index* work in a slightly different way to other indexing and abstracting services. Eugene Garfield, who started ISI, defines a citation index as 'an ordered list of references (cited works) in which each reference is followed by a list of the sources (citing works) which cite it'. Its main purpose is to lead the searcher from a key paper to others which have referred to that key paper, assuming that they will be relevant. It is published every two months with annual cumulations.

Excerpta Medica

Excerpta Medica Foundation and its associate, the publisher Elsevier, also publish a series of monthly or twice monthly printed bibliographies on selected medical topics. These are available as the *EMBASE* database.

Other bibliographies

There are also many specialised published bibliographic listings for particular areas in health and medicine. The British Library produces a series called *Healthcare Updates* which are either monthly or quarterly and cover topics from asthma to learning disabilities. These are inexpensive to subscribe to and keep healthcare professionals up to date with developments.

Electronic resources

Most bibliographies are now available electronically either locally through CD-ROM or on the Internet. Many libraries are switching from CD-ROM access to Internet access as the cost of local calls and Internet connections come down. It is perhaps interesting to note that searching has come full circle from the 1960s and 1970s when on-line searching was first made available to libraries. When on-line searching through various 'host' centres first became available, there was a worry that making this method of searching available in libraries would lead to huge telephone costs as readers tried the new searching techniques for themselves. This led to the whole idea of intermediary searching where the librarian did the searching for the reader and presented them with the results. There is a still a remnant of this thinking in libraries with the Internet, although this is now becoming less of a concern. Many end-users now access the Internet and free *Medline* for their searches. It should be noted, however, that *Medline* is the database and SilverPlatter, OVID and PubMed are just means of accessing the *Medline* database – this seems to cause some confusion among readers.

Medline via CD-ROM and the Internet

Medline is possibly the most famous medical bibliography in the world. Started in 1966 by the NLM, it was the electronic version of *Index Medicus* and was indexed using *MeSH* headings, which allowed for very controlled searching at the time. Techniques for accessing *Medline* have changed over the years. Originally tapes were supplied by the NLM and these were run on the host countries' computers – the host had to be a government department; the British Library took on this role in the UK and made *Medline* available via their BLAISE system. This changed in the 1970s and 1980s when a dial-up 'on-line' service direct to the NLM was offered and other host services were allowed to hold *Medline*. In the late 1980s access via CD-ROM became popular and in 1997 the NLM offered *Medline* free on the Internet via *PubMed* and *Internet Grateful Med*. *Medline*, as the electronic version of the printed *Index Medicus*, covers about 4000 journals and these remain roughly constant, with new journals being taken on and old ones dropped. The Board of Regents of the NLM decide on which titles should be included in *Medline* using various criteria such as timeliness and whether the journal is peer-reviewed.

Although the next section is about the various ways of searching *Medline*, it applies equally to the other electronic databases listed.

CD-ROM – OVID, SilverPlatter and the rest

There are two main suppliers of CD-ROM versions of *Medline* in the UK. These are SilverPlatter and OVID. SilverPlatter is the older of the two companies. Traditionally it would appear that NHS libraries favour OVID while higher education libraries favour SilverPlatter, although with consortium deals becoming the norm, that may change. Both offer very similar facilities but search in slightly different ways. CD-ROM has not yet been superseded by Internet versions even with 'free' *Medline* on the Internet. Reasons for this vary but libraries have invested in the infrastructure of CD-ROM, buying jukeboxes and RAID disk arrays, and many librarians prefer the interface of the CD-ROM to that on the Internet.

A disadvantage of CD-ROM is its currency. Most databases on CD-ROM are updated monthly but can still run several months behind. Most large databases also require more than one CD-ROM to contain them and updating on a regular basis can be difficult and time-consuming. On-line access through a host system or the Internet can make this a lot easier and the databases supplied this way tend to be much more up to date.

Two other suppliers who you may come across as well are EBSCO and Aries Knowledge Finder. EBSCO has *Comprehensive Medline* on CD-ROM, as well as a number of other biomedical databases, but many libraries will access databases through the EBSCOHost system on the Web. Aries Knowledge Finder is also popular with some sites in the UK.

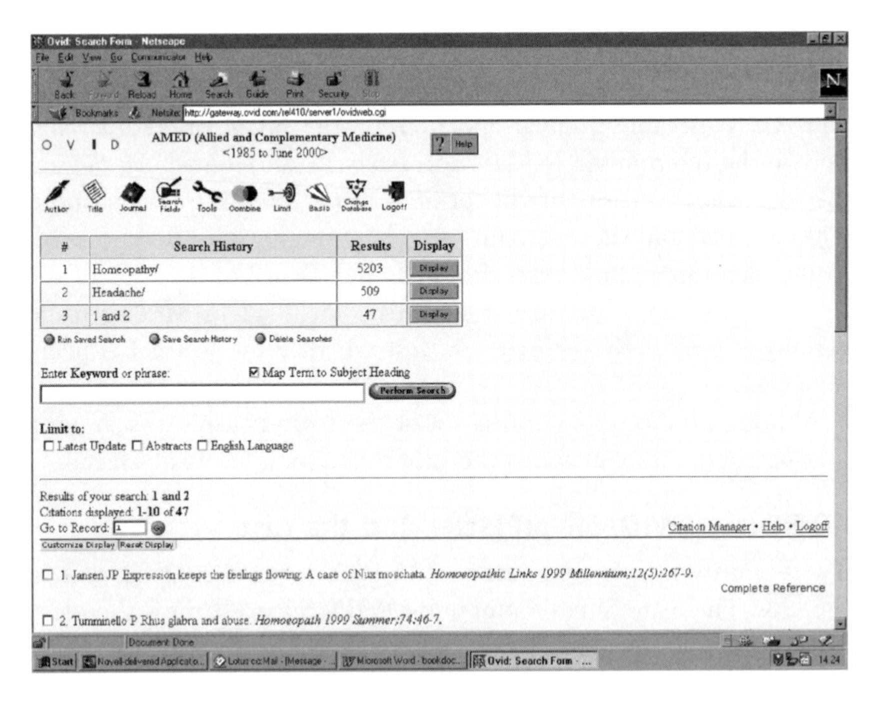

Figure 4.1 The OVID web interface

OVID versus SilverPlatter

Both versions offer different search interfaces to *Medline* and the other databases they provide. OVID has been favoured by many librarians because of its automatic mapping facility, although SilverPlatter also offers this in a slightly different form. On both systems you are presented with a search box into which you type your terms.

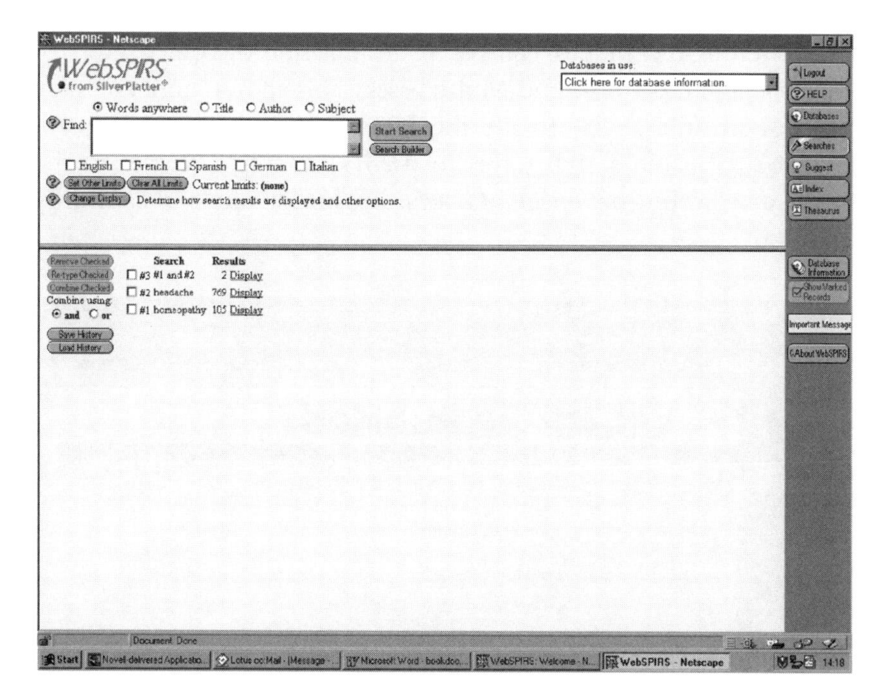

Figure 4.2 The *WebSpirs* interface from SilverPlatter

When you type in a search term, OVID maps to what it considers is the most appropriate *MeSH* heading for *Medline*, whereas Silver-Platter does the same through the 'suggest' button. Both versions have a complete copy of *MeSH* built in to the system (this is also true for the Internet versions), so the most appropriate *MeSH* term can be chosen. Both will allow you to combine search terms, using the number of the search statement, and then view your results in a variety of formats, either short format without abstract or long with abstract and *MeSH* headings. A printing or downloading facility is also offered but may depend on what the library holding the database will allow you to do.

Internet – *PubMed* and *Internet Grateful Med*

Since June 1997, *Medline* and the other NLM databases have been made freely available on the Internet. *PubMed* (http://www.ncbi.nlm.nih.gov:80/entrez/query.fcgi) is the NLM's search service that provides access to over 11 million citations in *Medline*, *PreMEDLINE* and other related databases, with links to participating on-line journals. *PubMed* is aimed at the novice searcher, although new features have been added to allow complex Boolean searches (*see* Searching techniques). *Internet Grateful Med* is the other interface for *Medline* and the other NLM databases. This allows more complex searches and the ability to use the *Unified Medical Language System* (*UMLS*) to match search terms to *MeSH* headings. However, the NLM may well drop *Internet Grateful Med* in favour of *PubMed* by mid-2001.

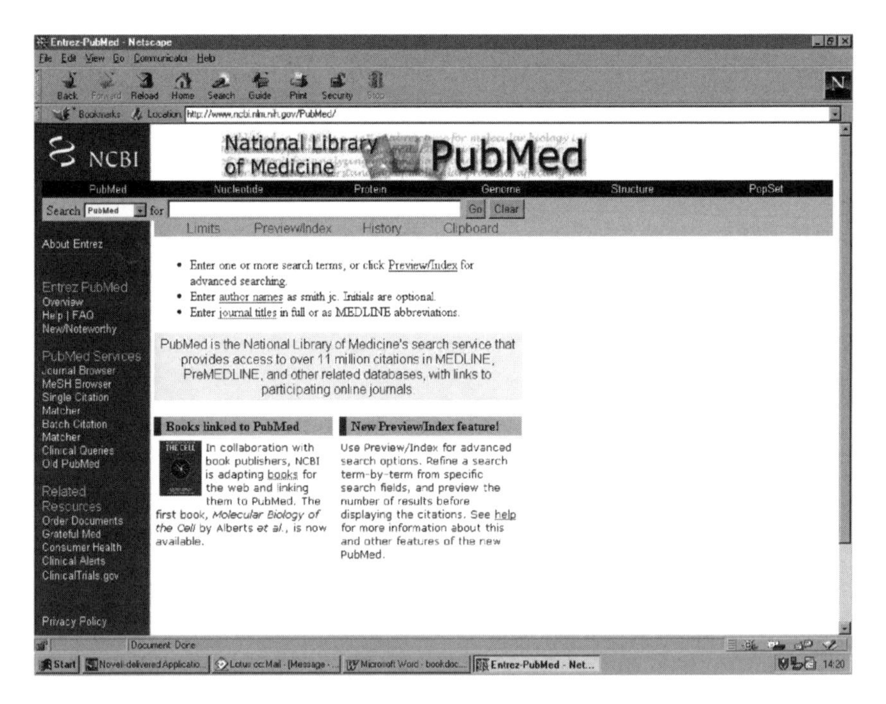

Figure 4.3 The *PubMed* search interface from the NLM

Other free Internet providers

There are a number of other Web-based hosts that offer *Medline* and various other NLM databases free of charge. *OMNI* (*see below*) offers a listing of these on its website. These include:

- *BioMedNet* – http://www.bmn.com/
  BioMedNet is owned by Elsevier Science and is the website for biological medical researchers. *BioMedNet* allows you to search *Medline* and the *Swiss-Prot* database (a protein sequence database), which is free, and members can search all of *BioMedNet* without charge. There is also a daily news update feature and *HMS Beagle*, a free magazine. Links to the British Library DSC allow you to order documents at a cost, and viewing full-text articles from publishers often requires payment or a subscription.
- *Healthworks* – http://www.healthworks.co.uk/
  Healthworks is a UK-based company that offers free *Medline* and a daily news feed as well as other useful links and information.

Online hosts

Although searching *Medline* and other databases on on-line hosts using a text-based command language is becoming less popular, it is still a way of accessing a large number of databases and allows cross-database searching and de-duplication of results. The rise of the Internet has resulted in many of the traditional on-line hosts offering a web interface to search the databases that they make available. The main on-line hosts are Datastar and Dialog, which are both owned by The Dialog Corporation (www.dialog.com) – DataStar is a European host while Dialog is mainly US-based, but with the World Wide Web these geographical limitations are seen as meaningless. Other hosts include the German host DIMDI (Deutsches Institut für Medizinische Dokumentation und Information), which makes a large number of databases available and has a web interface, and the European Information Network Services (EINS – http://www.eins.org/), a consortium of European hosts including DIMDI, which makes a wide range of scientific databases available to researchers. None of these hosts is free and all attract a charge for searching, so some competency in searching and preparation before actually 'going on-line' is necessary to keep costs down.

OVID, SilverPlatter, EBSCO and Aries also provide web access to their databases on a subscription basis, with links to document supply features and full-text electronic journals where they are available. OVID also provides the *Core Biomedical Collection* of full-text electronic journals, which are some of the most popular journals made available to subscribers.

Another service that is becoming more popular is HCN's MIRON system, which provides access to many biomedical databases including *Medline*, *CINAHL* and *AMED*.

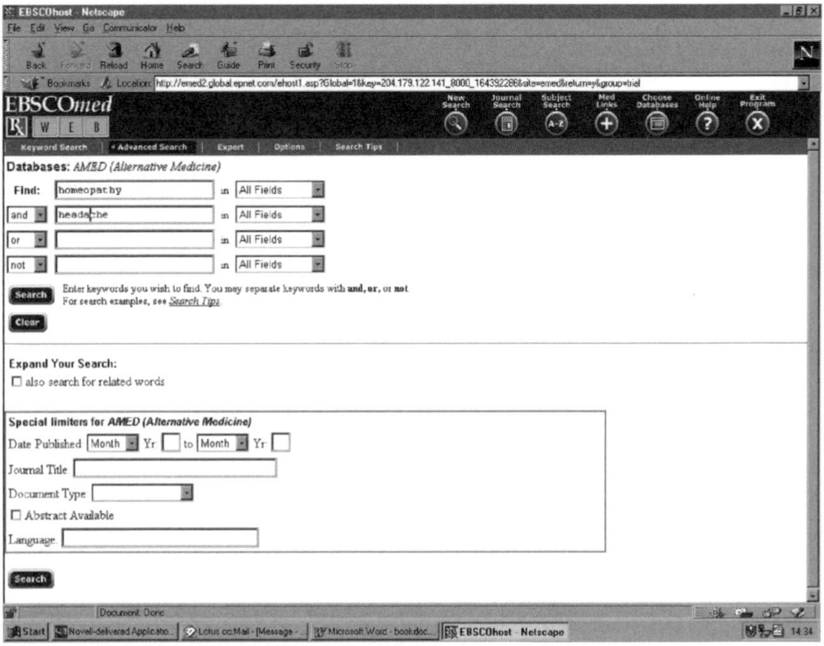

Figure 4.4 The EBSCO*med* advanced search interface

Bath Information and Data Service (BIDS) – http://www.bids.ac.uk/

BIDS is a name you will come across regularly in the higher education sector. *BIDS* is probably the best-known and most widely used bibliographic service for the academic community in the UK. It also provides access to a full-text journals service, around 2500 full-text electronic journals, both directly and also through links from database search results. Launched in 1991, *BIDS* is believed to have been a world first – a national service providing widespread network access to commercially supplied bibliographic databases, free at the point of delivery.

BIDS is hosted by the University of Bath and performs an important role in the information strategy of the Joint Information Systems Committee of the Higher Education Funding Councils

(JISC). It is one of three data centres funded by the JISC, along with MIMAS (located at Manchester University) and EDINA (located at Edinburgh University).

The University of Bath also hosts the other JISC-funded services: CHEST, NISS, and UKOLN.

EMBASE

EMBASE is produced by Elsevier Scientific Publications and is the electronic version of the *Excerpta Medica* published abstracts on various topics (mentioned in the previous section). *EMBASE* also has a thesaurus of terms called EMTREE, which is also available as a separate paper publication. *EMBASE* indexes about the same number of journals as *Medline*, 3800, but there is only about 30–40% overlap and *EMBASE* is particularly strong in the pharmaceutical area. It is really the other major medical bibliography and for a really complete search should be searched alongside *Medline*. It is not as common in libraries as *Medline*, although there are moves in place, with consortium buying, to rectify the situation. It is available on CD-ROM and the Internet from OVID, SilverPlatter and EBSCO.

CINAHL

The *Cumulative Index of Nursing and Allied Health Literature* (*CINAHL*) is produced by CINAHL Information Systems in Glendale, California. It covers the nursing and allied health disciplines, which include the therapies such as physiotherapy and occupational therapy, as well as laboratory technology and nutrition. They index more than 1100 journals. They also include books and pamphlets, dissertations, proceedings, standards and software. Original documents include drug records, accreditation, legal cases and clinical innovation. Some selected full-text material is also included. The database is available from a number of suppliers, on-line through Dialog and DataStar and on CD-ROM through OVID, SilverPlatter and EBSCO.

British Nursing Index (*BNI*)

The *British Nursing Index* is produced by the Royal College of Nursing and the University of Bournemouth with Poole Hospital NHS Trust. It indexes journal articles from all the major British nursing and midwifery titles and other English-language titles, over

200 journals in total. The topics covered include all aspects of nursing and some information on alternative therapies. It is available on CD-ROM from SilverPlatter and by password on the Internet (www.bni.org.uk).

Health Management Information Consortium (HMIC)

HMIC covers health management information both in the UK and internationally. It is a collection of three bibliographic databases – The Department of Health's database, which is also available separately as *DHData* on DataStar, the *King's Fund* database and *HELMIS*, formerly produced by the Nuffield Institute for Health but no longer available. The CD-ROM and web versions are available from SilverPlatter.

Allied and Complementary Medicine Database (*AMED*)

AMED is produced by the British Library's Health Care Information Service and covers the areas of complementary medicine, physiotherapy, occupational therapy, rehabilitation medicine, palliative care, podiatry, and speech and language therapy. Its coverage extends back to 1985, when the database was started due to the lack of coverage of these topics on *Medline*. It has a thesaurus of terms based on *MeSH* and since 1993 has included short abstracts. It is available as print, and on CD-ROM through SilverPlatter and OVID as well as on the Web via EBSCO*Med*.

Applied Social Science Index and Abstracts (*ASSIA*)

ASSIA covers the areas of the social sciences, which include geriatrics, child abuse, and NHS reforms and management. It indexes about 550 journals and each record includes a short abstract. A subset, *ASSIA Health*, has been produced by SilverPlatter in association with HCN. It is available on Dialog and DataStar and the publisher, Bowker-Saur, produces its own CD-ROM version of the main *ASSIA* database.

PsycINFO and *PsycLIT*

The *PsycINFO* database corresponds to the printed *Psychological Abstracts* produced by the American Psychological Association (APA), which covers the international literature on psychology and psychiatry from 1887. It indexes more than 1400 international journals and about 57 000 references are added annually. *PsycINFO* is available on-line through DataStar, Dialog and DIMDI, but subsets are available on CD-ROM. *PsycLIT* is a subset dealing with the academic and professional literature on psychology, and *CLINPsyc* is a subset dealing with medical and clinical psychology; both are available via OVID, SilverPlatter and EBSCO Publishing. It is possible that the APA will, in future, withdraw the subsets in favour of libraries taking the whole *PsycINFO* database.

The above are probably the major databases that will be available in any health library but there is far more specialised data available to the researcher or healthcare professional. A few other databases may be worth mentioning for more in-depth searching.

Health Economic Evaluations Database (*HEED*)

HEED is produced by the Office for Health Economics and contains information on cost-effectiveness of medicine and other treatments. It contains information on more than 15 000 economic evaluations, over half of which have been reviewed by a panel of experts. About 200 fully reviewed articles are added each month. They are selected from on-line databases and the leading journals but some unpublished material is also included. *HEED* is available for a yearly subscription.

NHS Health database

The database contains three modules which can be used together or separately. One module contains health authority commissioning plans, public health reports and service reviews. The Primary Care Group module contains details from PCGs and the 'Provider' module contains trust annual reports and service plans. The database is available on CD-ROM and is produced by Blackwell Masters Ltd and the NHS Confederation.

OECD Health Data

OECD Health Data is a useful tool for comparing health data between OECD (Organization for Economic Cooperation and Development) member countries. It includes information such as health status, financing, resources and the market. You can sample the data at www.oecd.org/els/health/software. It is available as a CD-ROM on subscription.

Other NLM databases

The NLM also produces a number of bibliographic databases on specific topics, for example *AIDSLINE*, which covers the area of HIV/AIDS, and *CANCERLIT*, which covers cancer. A list of these databases is available from the NLM website (www.nlm.nih.gov) and they are currently searchable through *Internet Grateful Med* (http://igm.nlm.nih.gov). Plans for the amalgamation of all of these databases into one huge database are under way and this will be searchable using the *PubMed* interface. Many are currently available through on-line hosts such as Dialog and DIMDI, and CD-ROMs exist of some of the more useful ones.

Toxicology databases

It is worth mentioning two sources for toxicology information as they are both provided by the NLM. *TOXLINE* is the bibliographic database which includes references going back to 1965, with some older key references. It contains references gleaned from *Medline, BIOSIS* and several US government publications from agencies such as NIOSH (National Institute of Occupational Safety and Health) and the EPA (Environmental Protection Agency). The other collection of databases is called *TOXNET*, and it contains pure data about the toxicity levels of chemical and biological substances. *TOXLINE* and the constituent databases of *TOXNET* are available through various on-line hosts such as Dialog and DIMDI. They are both available on the Web through the NLM's Specialized Information Services home page (http://sis.nlm.nih.gov/tehip.cfm) and *TOXLINE* can be subscribed to on SilverPlatter CD-ROM.

Keeping up to date

For keeping really current in your subject, you need to use a 'current awareness service'. These databases are not indexed in great depth as currency is their main aim and the indexing of articles takes time. Usually you can search by a keyword in the title or by author or journal title. *Current Contents* is also available as a print version (*see* Chapter 3).

Infotrieve – http://www3.infotrieve.com/medline/infotrieve

Infotrieve offer a free web-based service for current awareness using the *Medline* database. You can set up your search using an easy, intuitive web form and the search is run every time the database is updated. It is easy to define a highly sophisticated search and to use such refinements as limits and age groups.

Mindit – http://mindit.netmind.com

This is a free service which alerts you every time a website that you are interested in is changed. It could be useful on sites that give details of grants, etc. An e-mail arrives every time the sites you choose are updated.

Inside – http://www.bl.uk/inside

Inside is the British Library's current awareness product. The contents pages of 21 000 of the most requested journals are keyed into a database which is updated regularly. The database is particularly strong on the science, technology and medical areas, and journals such as the *BMJ* are added to the database within a couple of days of receipt. In addition to the searching capabilities, you can also order documents from the British Library's collection at a cost which includes a copyright fee. *Inside Alerts* offers a selected profile of journal titles to be run against the *Inside* database and the contents pages of those journals are delivered directly to the user's e-mail address.

Current Contents

Current Contents is also available electronically as a disk or on-line through the DataStar and Dialog host systems. Both OVID and SilverPlatter have a CD-ROM. You can also get *Current Contents* through the ISI's *Web of Science*. For more detail on *Current Contents* *see* page 29.

Web of Science – http://www.isinet.com/

The *Web of Science* is the Internet version of the citation indexes produced by ISI – *see* Science Citation Index in the previous section. *Web of Science* contains the following databases:

- *Science Citation Index Expanded with Cited References and Author Abstracts (1981–)*
- *Social Science Citation Index Expanded with Cited References and Author Abstracts (1981–)*
- *Arts & Humanities Citation Index with Cited References (1981–).*

It also gives access to the *Index to Scientific and Technical Proceedings (ISTP) (1990–)*, which indexes the published literature of the most significant conferences, symposia, seminars, colloquia workshops and conventions in a wide range of disciplines in science and technology.

In addition, other products are available for an extra charge: these include *Current Contents Connect* (*CCC*), which is a current awareness database that includes information in the fields of science, social science, technology, and arts and humanities. The latest version features profile-based alerting that gives users the ability to create and manage a set number of alerts that will run against the *Current Contents* data. Once a week, the results are automatically forwarded to a specified e-mail address.

The *Current Contents* titles included are:

- *Life Sciences with Author Abstracts*
- *Clinical Medicine with Author Abstracts*
- *Agriculture, Biology & Environmental Sciences with Author Abstracts*
- *Engineering, Computing & Technology with Author Abstracts*
- *Physical, Chemical & Earth Sciences with Author Abstracts*
- *Social & Behavioral Sciences with Author Abstracts*
- *Arts & Humanities (no Author Abstracts available).*

Also on *Web of Science* are the *Journal Citation Reports* (*JCR*), which are a comprehensive, and unique resource for journal evaluation, using citation data drawn from over 8400 scholarly and technical journals worldwide. Coverage is both multidisciplinary and international, and incorporates journals from over 3000 publishers in 60 nations.

The *JCR* is the only source of citation data on journals and includes virtually all specialities in the areas of science, technology and the social sciences. *JCR Web* shows the relationship between citing and cited journals. *JCR Web* is available annually in two editions:

- *Science Edition*, which contains data from roughly 5000 journals in the areas of science and technology
- *Social Sciences Edition*, which contains data from roughly 1500 journals in the social sciences.

Due to an agreement with CHEST (Combined Higher Education Software Team), which purchases databases and software for the higher education sector in the UK, you will find *Web of Science* in most university libraries and some of the larger NHS trust libraries.

Patient information

Although this book is aimed at those using health libraries, it is worth mentioning a couple of useful sites for information aimed at patients rather than healthcare professionals as, in the course of your career, it may be useful to know where to go for such information. You will find that many NHS libraries already provide access to patients and have a range of materials for their use. A look at consumer health information is also included in Chapter 9, as it is an area which is growing and will have a great deal of influence in the future.

Helpbox

Helpbox is produced by the Help for Health Trust in Winchester. It is a computerised database which is made available on disk and runs under the Microsoft Windows operating system. It contains three files and can be edited to add local information. The data contained includes self-help group addresses, leaflets and books.

Medline Plus – http://medlineplus.gov/

Medline Plus is another database available from the NLM. It provides access to extensive information about specific diseases and conditions and also has links to consumer health information from the NIH, dictionaries, lists of hospitals and physicians, health information in Spanish and other languages, and clinical trials.

Healthfinder – http://www.healthfinder.gov/

Healthfinder is a free gateway to consumer health and human services information developed by the US Department of Health and Human Services. It contains selected on-line publications, clearing-houses, databases, websites, and support and self-help groups, as well as the government agencies and not-for-profit organisations that produce information for the public. It was launched in April 1997 and served Internet users over 1.7 million times in its first year on-line.

NHS Direct Online – http://www.nhsdirect.nhs.uk/

NHS Direct Online is the web version of the NHS Direct telephone triage service. It makes information available for patients about the NHS, as well as simple guides to conditions and treatments which can be administered at home.

Other similar services are offered by *doctors.net* (www.doctors.net), *Surgery Door* (http://www.surgerydoor.co.uk) and *NetDoctor*, which is an independent medical site at (http://www.netdoctor.co.uk).

Searching techniques

This can only be a basic guide to searching electronic databases – your local librarian should be able to help with the more detailed searching techniques that can be used with each database. As a start you will find that the best way to search is to break down your query into its separate topics. The examples given below can be run on most systems, whether on CD-ROM, on-line or on the Net – the only difference would be the look of the interface.

You will find that most of the database interfaces now run under a graphical user interface (GUI) such as Microsoft Windows or the Apple Macintosh interface, depending on which system your library favours. The search screen will therefore have a list of commands on a menu bar across the top of the screen and a search box where you can enter your search terms. Under this will be some sort of results box which will tell you how many items you have retrieved for each term you entered and these will be given a 'search statement' number, for example:

1: Homeopathy	2000
2: Headache	500
3: 1 & 2	10

In the example above we have looked for the use of homeopathy in headaches. We have typed in homeopathy and headache, and the system has assigned the search statement numbers 1 and 2 to the two search terms. The system has then combined the two terms to bring up a third result with both terms included. This introduces the concept of Boolean logic which you may hear librarians talking about. The three statements most commonly used are AND, OR,

NOT – and these can be used to give differing results in a search. For example, HOMEOPATHY *and* HEADACHE would find articles which include both the terms 'homeopathy' and 'headache'. HOMEOPATHY *or* HEADACHE would retrieve more articles, as it is looking for the two terms and so would recover articles containing the word 'homeopathy' or the word 'headache'. HOMEOPATHY *not* HEADACHE would locate articles about homeopathy but not those where the word 'headache' also appears.

By assigning search statement numbers, the user can build up complicated searches, e.g. 1 and 2 not 3, without having to type the terms in again, which can be useful when you get on to your 25th search term!

The user can also use brackets to build even more complicated search statements, e.g. (HOMEOPATHY or ACUPUNCTURE) not (HEADACHE or ASTHMA) would retrieve terms which were on homeopathy or acupuncture but not where those articles contained the words 'asthma' or 'headache'.

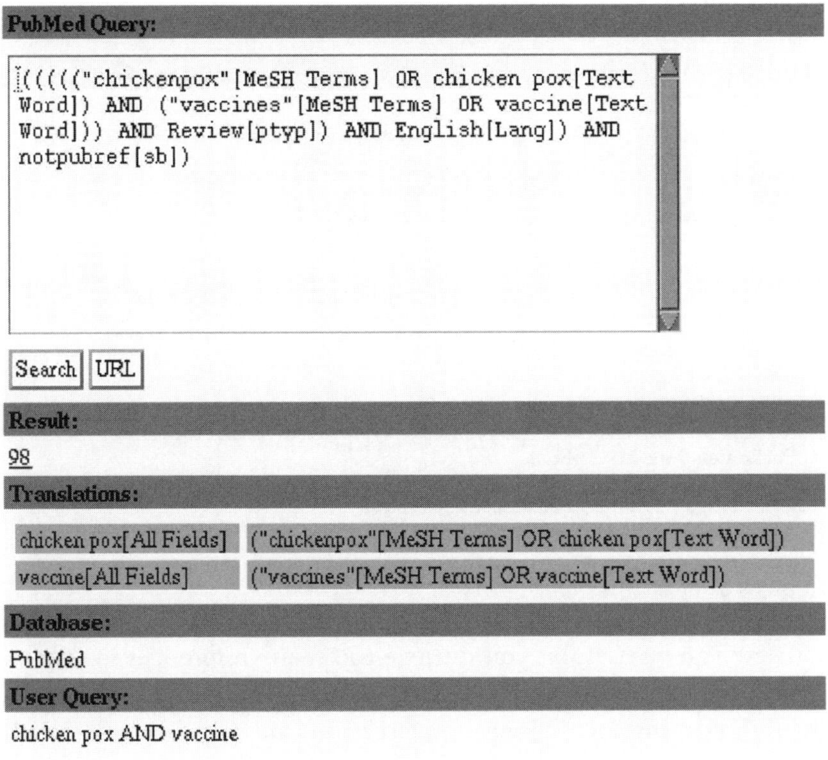

PubMed Query:

```
(((((("chickenpox"[MeSH Terms] OR chicken pox[Text
Word]) AND ("vaccines"[MeSH Terms] OR vaccine[Text
Word])) AND Review[ptyp]) AND English[Lang]) AND
notpubref[sb])
```

Search URL

Result:

98

Translations:

chicken pox[All Fields]	("chickenpox"[MeSH Terms] OR chicken pox[Text Word])
vaccine[All Fields]	("vaccines"[MeSH Terms] OR vaccine[Text Word])

Database:

PubMed

User Query:

chicken pox AND vaccine

Figure 4.5 A Boolean search in *PubMed*

Truncation is also a useful tool for searching. For example, CHILD$ would retrieve 'child' or 'children' – the $ symbol just substitutes a number of letters. The $, # or colon signs are popular and used in many systems – the help files for the system should be able to guide you as to the correct symbol. It is also worth noting that too much truncation can lead to interesting results so that CH$ would locate 'child' or 'children' but also 'chilli', 'chestnut', etc.

It should also be noted that all systems will have a series of stopwords which you should avoid using in your searches. These are fairly common and consist of words such as 'and', 'the', 'but', etc.

Most systems will also allow you to impose limits on your search. These include:

- human or animal
- age ranges, e.g. 0–10, 10–20, or adolescent, middle-aged, elderly
- publication type, e.g. review, guideline, etc.
- language of publication, e.g. English or French, etc.
- date ranges, e.g. 1990–99.

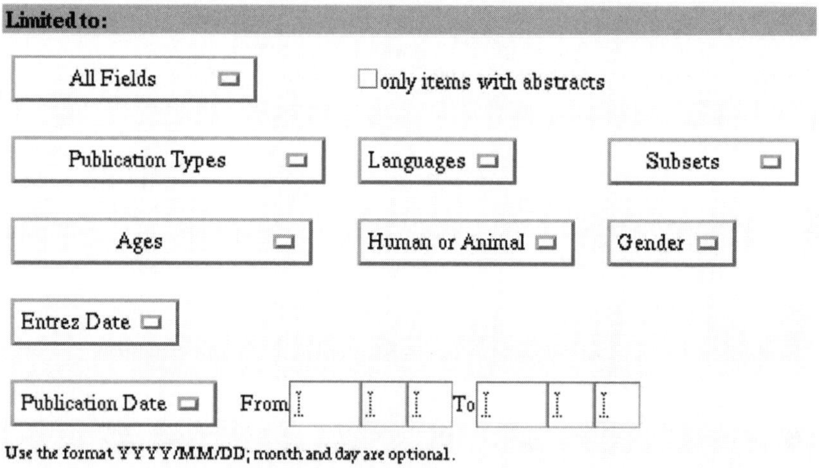

Figure 4.6 The limit feature in *PubMed*

These can be useful if you retrieve too many references in the first place. Age ranges are preferred if searching for articles about the elderly. For instance, doing a search on the word 'aged' would retrieve articles with titles including the word 'aged', i.e. patients *aged* between 10 and 20. Publication type can be useful for an overview of a subject, e.g. if you are searching for asthma and retrieve thousands of references, by using the 'review' publication type you will retrieve only articles that are reviews of the topic. It is also worth remembering that certain publications specialise in reviews only, e.g. the *Annual Reviews* series or the *Clinics of North America* series. Reviews can also be biased towards the author's point of view so it may be worth retrieving more than one review. A course on 'critical appraisal' skills might be useful if you are going to be recovering a lot of literature for a project.

Medline also provides 'subheadings' which are listed in the printed *MeSH* and also on most of the electronic versions of the database. Subheadings are applied to each section of *MeSH* – for instance the 'C LIST', which is the section for general diseases, includes the following:

BL /blood	EP /epidemiology	PX /psychology
CF /cerebrospinal fluid	ET /etiology	RA /radiography
CI /chemical industry	GE /genetics	RH /rehabilitation
CL /classification	HI /history	RI /radionuclide
CN /congenital	IM /immunology	RT /radiotherapy
CO /complications	ME /metabolism	SU /surgery
DH /diet therapy	MI /microbiology	TH /therapy
DI /diagnosis	MO /mortality	UR /urine
DT /drug therapy	NU /nursing	US /ultrasonography
EC /economics	PA /pathology	VE /veterinary
EH /ethnology	PC /prevention	VI /virology
EM /embryology	PP /physiopathology	
EN /enzymology	PS /parasitology	

The two-letter tag can be added to your search term as a sort of qualifier, so drug terms will allow you to add 'AE' for adverse effects or 'PO' for poisoning. As a practical example, in *Internet Grateful Med* (http://igm.nlm.nih.gov) when you type a term into one of the search boxes and click on the 'find related' button, the browser takes you to the most appropriate *MeSH* term. If you select this in the tick box, the system then allows you to assign a subheading to make that search more specific and transfers the search term back to the search screen.

Finding 'grey' literature, including official publications

'Grey' literature is usually classified as that material that does not have an ISBN or ISSN. It includes technical reports, official publications and report materials. It can also contain a lot of useful information, including statistics and research findings, but it is always difficult to track down in catalogues. It may also be difficult to collect, unless the publisher deposits the publication with a legal deposit library. One database that tries to list grey literature is *SIGLE*.

System for Information on Grey Literature In Europe (SIGLE)

SIGLE is produced by the EAGLE consortium – the British Library is the UK partner – and covers grey literature from 1980 to date. It provides access to records for reports and other grey literature in all subject areas produced in Europe. The database contains records from nine European countries, along with some of the R&D material produced by the Commission of the European Communities. The majority of material cited is in English, and those items indicated as being held at the British Library DSC can be ordered on-line. Many documents cited as being from other sources may also be available from DSC. The file is updated monthly and is currently available on-line on BLAISE-LINE from the British Library and on CD-ROM from SilverPlatter.

For official publications the following two sites are a mine of information and are a good place to start.

- **The Stationery Office – http://www.official-documents.co.uk/**
  The Stationery Office (formerly Her Majesty's Stationery Office – HMSO) has a very comprehensive website which lists all available governmental publications. They also publish daily, weekly and monthly lists of government publications in print to which some health libraries will subscribe.
- **The Department of Health – http://www.doh.gov.uk/**
  The Department of Health (DoH) site has grown in importance and is now one of the major ways for finding out about the DoH, the NHS and the publications they produce. Two catalogues of publications, *Circulars on the Net* (*COIN*) and *Publications on the*

Internet (*POINT*) list circulars and publications respectively. A subject search, however, is not recommended as the whole site is searched, so you need to be able to start from a point where you know the circular number or the publication title. That said, it is a useful tool for tracking down and printing copies of DoH circulars.

Theses and dissertations

Based on the holdings of the National Reports Collection at the British Library DSC, *British Reports, Translation and Theses* (*BRTT*) is a listing of newly published reports, technical papers and dissertations produced by non-commercial publishers such as research institutions, private and public sector organisations, charities and action groups. English translations of foreign-language reports and doctoral theses are also included. All subject areas are covered. It is published monthly, with a microfiche index of cumulated key terms, authors and report numbers which is supplied quarterly, and is available on subscription.

The *Index to Theses accepted for higher degrees by the Universities of Great Britain and Ireland* has been available as a print subscription for a number of years and was originally produced by ASLIB (Association of Libraries and Information Bureaux). However, the index is now available on the Web at http://www.theses.com/. The database covers theses accepted from 1970 to 1999, covering all of volumes 21 to 48 and parts 1 to 3 of volume 49 of the equivalent print publication *Index to Theses*.

Further reading

Core Research Ltd (1999) *Core Resources of Healthcare Information*. Alton, Hampshire.

Tyrrell S (1999) *Using the Internet in Healthcare. Harnessing Health Information Series No.2*. Radcliffe Medical Press, Oxford.

Wyatt J (1991) Use and sources of medical knowledge. *Lancet*. **338**(8779): 1368–73.

5 The reference enquiry

Directories and other reference works of use

There is a large number of directories that are relevant to the health arena, so I shall deal only with the ones that I have found to be of most use when looking for details of people or companies.

Dictionaries and other 'word' books

There are three main medical dictionaries that you may well find in the medical library:

- Macpherson G (1999) *Black's Medical Dictionary* (39e). A & C Black, London. This is the 'English' dictionary and is very comprehensive, including brief biographical notes, eponyms and abbreviations.
- Dorland WAN (2000) *Dorland's Illustrated Medical Dictionary* (29e). WB Saunders, Philadelphia. Accomplished and up to date but with American spellings; a pocket version is also available.
- Stedman TL *et al.* (2000) *Stedman's Medical Dictionary*. Lippincott, Williams and Wilkins, Philadelphia and London (27e). A wide-ranging standard dictionary which includes brief biographies and is also available on CD-ROM for integration with word-processing packages.

For syndromes and eponymic diseases, the following two books are by far the best and most comprehensive:

- Jablonski S (1991) *Jablonski's Dictionary of Syndromes and Eponymic Diseases* (7e). Krieger, Malabar, FL.
- Magalini SI (*c.* 1997) *Dictionary of Medical Syndromes* (4e). Lippincott-Raven, Philadelphia.

Medical quotations

For medical quotations, I would look up:

- Strauss MB (1968). *Familiar Medical Quotations*. Little Brown, Boston. Quotations are arranged by subject, and dates of birth and death are given. However, few original sources are given.

Directories

Directories are amazingly useful sources of addresses and basic information about a wide range of topics. There are literally hundreds of directories, so I have given only the most useful ones here.

- The *Medical Register* is the official list of registered doctors in the UK. It comes in three volumes and is produced annually. Most health libraries will have a copy.
- The *Medical Directory,* produced annually by FT Healthcare, is the unofficial list of doctors and is compiled from questionnaires. It contains details of over 132 000 practitioners and lists of NHS trusts and independent hospitals. There is also now a CD-ROM version which contains more information and allows material to be downloaded.
- The Institute of Health Service Managers *IHSM Hospital and Health Services Yearbook*, published annually by FT Healthcare, contains a wealth of information on NHS trusts and independent hospitals, publications and suppliers, and a comprehensive bibliography of useful publications. It is also now available as a CD-ROM which can be used to create mailing label lists.
- The publisher Binleys also produces a series of very useful directories covering lists of trusts and managers as well as PCGs. Most NHS libraries will have either the IHSM publication or the Binleys publications. Either can be used to get more details about addresses and NHS and private establishments.
- The *NHS Handbook* is also useful as it provides a comprehensive description of the health service structure as well as the latest policy developments and up-to-date facts and figures. It also includes a full listing of NHS trusts and health authorities and useful chapters about developments in the NHS. It is published annually by the NHS Confederation.

University listings

The *World of Learning* is produced annually by Europa Publications in London and is a listing of educational, scientific and cultural establishments around the world. It includes universities and colleges, academies, research institutes, libraries and museums, all arranged alphabetically by country with an index of institutions. It is useful for finding out about staff details.

The *Commonwealth Universities Yearbook* is similar to the *World of Learning* and includes data on the universities of the Commonwealth. It gives names and addresses of staff, admission requirements and affiliations. It is produced annually by the Association of Commonwealth Universities in London.

A Guide to Postgraduate Degrees, Diplomas and Courses in Medicine (and there is also one for dentistry) is compiled annually by the Council for Postgraduate Medical Education in England and Wales on behalf of the three Councils of the United Kingdom. It has been available since 1983.

Grants and charities

When looking for sources of funding there are two major directories which are updated annually and which are fairly comprehensive. They are:

Charities Aid Foundation: the directory of grant making trusts (CAF Publications, Tonbridge, Kent) is published annually, as is *The Grants Register* (Macmillan, London and Basingstoke).

In the US there is the *Directory of Biomedical and Health Care Grants* published by Oryx Press, Phoenix, Arizona.

Private healthcare

When it comes to details of private healthcare and independent hospitals, the most useful directory that is published annually is *Laing's Review of Private Healthcare*, Laing and Buisson, London. It includes short articles about items of interest as well as a comprehensive listing of all private health establishments and their staff.

Associations and professional bodies

CBD, based in Beckenham in Kent, produce a number of useful directories that list organisations and associations. The two of most use are: *Directory of British Associations & Associations in Ireland* and the *Directory of European Medical Organisations*. Both are updated regularly and list most of the associations with name, address, telephone and fax number, and organisation details.

Conferences

To find details of conferences, the best tool is the *Index to Conference Proceedings* which was produced by the British Library until 1988 when Bowker-Saur took over production. It lists all conferences for which the British Library has received the proceedings. The library in turn indexes conference proceedings on its *Inside* product (*see above*).

There are also some websites that list forthcoming conferences; a particularly useful site is at http://www.nlm.nih.gov/services/medmeet.html.

Vital statistics

Most healthcare professionals need to track down vital statistics at some time in their career. The list below shows some of the more useful publications that can help with statistical enquiries.

- The WHO has published its *World Health Statistics Annual* each year since 1952. It contains life tables, morbidity and mortality rates for most countries of the world in both English and French. The WHO website gives users access to its Statistical Information Service (WHOSIS) and is available at http://www.who.int/.
- The Stationery Office publishes the *Annual Abstract of Statistics* which is compiled by the Office for National Statistics (ONS) in London. This publication covers more than health statistics but gives a good overview of the UK in numbers and covers about ten years of data, so comparisons can be made. It includes population and vital statistics, mortality rates by age and cause, life tables and infectious disease notifications.
- ONS, formerly the Office of Population Censuses and Surveys (OPCS), produces a lot of useful health information, much of which is available through its website http://www.ons.gov.uk. Most of the material is derived from the national registration system for births and deaths and the ONS's systems for notification of congenital abnormalities and infectious diseases. It also carries out work on behalf of the DoH and the Health Development Agency (formerly the Health Education Authority).
- Since 1999, The Stationery Office has produced the *Health*

Statistics Quarterly, which is a source of information on all aspects of health.

- The DoH produces *On the State of the Public Health*, which is the annual report of the Chief Medical Officer. It gives some statistical data but is particularly useful for topics of current interest.
- A good way of finding out about UK official statistics on health and healthcare is the companion volume in the *Harnessing Health Information* series. Leadbeter D (ed) (2000) *Harnessing Official Statistics*, Radcliffe Medical Press, Oxford, identifies the principal types of health statistics and their sources, followed by chapters on their main applications, such as health outcomes analyses.
- *Medistat: world medical market analysis* (MDIS Publications, Chichester) is a very interesting publication and is available as a loose-leaf print version which is regularly updated or as a CD-ROM. It lists details of the health expenditure as GDP (gross domestic product), hospital addresses, medical device companies and pharmaceutical companies for all countries of the world, and is a really useful directory.

Pharmaceutical literature

The tracking down of information in the pharmaceutical field is a whole topic in itself. Some of the more useful directories and information sources are given below.

- The most useful pharmacopoeia is *Martindale, the extra pharmacopoeia* (31e), edited by James EF Reynolds, deputy editor Kathleen Parfitt, assistant editors Anne V Parsons and Sean C Sweetman, Royal Pharmaceutical Society, London, 1996. *Martindale* contains chapters on the major drug types. A general description of the drug type is given, followed by details of each drug, including trade names, dosage, adverse effects and references. *Martindale* is available on CD-ROM and is searchable online through Dialog.
- *British Pharmacopoeia 2000* (now with accompanying CD-ROM), The Stationery Office, London. This is the accepted legal standard in Britain and the Commonwealth for the drugs included in it. Publication is on the recommendation of the Medicines Commission. The standards laid down in the *European Pharmacopoeia* are largely becoming the standards in Britain.

- *British Herbal Pharmacopoeia* (4e), British Herbal Medicine Association, 1996, is the herbal equivalent of the *British Pharmacopoeia*, and the *British Homeopathic Pharmacopoeia* (2e), British Association of Homeopathic Manufacturers, Rutland, 1999, is the homeopathic equivalent.
- The Association of British Pharmaceutical Industries produces the *Compendium of Data Sheets and Summaries of Product Characteristics* (aka the *Data Sheet Compendium*) which is sent free each year to practitioners and pharmacists. It contains text for the summaries of product descriptions, approved by the Medicines Agency, for most of the medicines available in the UK. The new electronic version is available on the Web at http://emc.vhn.net/ and is divided into three categories – one for healthcare professionals, one for pharmaceutical companies and one for the general public. Users need to register to use the site but there are no charges for doing this.
- The most frequently consulted drug text is probably the *British National Formulary*, which is published every six months, and most doctors carry a copy around with them in their pockets. It is produced jointly by the Royal Pharmaceutical Society and the BMA and is also available as the electronic *BNF* (*e-BNF*) on CD-ROM with the *Drug and Therapeutics Bulletin*, and the *MeReC Bulletin*, which lists new medicines.
- The *Monthly Index of Medical Specialties* (*MIMS*) is written by independent experts and is designed as a prescribing guide for GPs. Information is written in a strictly controlled format which includes prescription-only medicine as well as some over-the-counter products if they have been approved by the Advisory Committee on Borderline Substances. A version is now available on CD-ROM.
- *The Merck Index: an encyclopedia of chemicals, drugs, and biologicals* (12e) (edited by Susan Budavari), Merck Research Laboratories, Whitehouse Station, NJ, 1999, also available as a CD-ROM with additional monographs, contains a series of monographs on drugs and other biological substances. It is now available as an on-line database through Dialog and STN (another European host) covering some 10 000 records. Each record contains systematic, generic, trivial and product names for a compound plus its CAS registry number, manufacturer, distributor, toxicity and usage. It

has bibliographic citations for each compound where these are relevant.

- For the adverse effects of drugs, the best information can be found in both *Meyler's Side Effects of Drugs* (Excerpta Medica, Amsterdam and Oxford, 1975) and *Side Effects of Drugs Annual* (edited by MNG Dukes *et al.*). These two combined form the database *SEDBASE*, which is available on-line from Datastar and Dialog, and are complete up to 1995. The database covers information on more than 50 000 drug side-effects and over 4000 drug interactions.
- The *Chemist and Druggist* is a monthly publication which is aimed at pharmacists and lists both drugs and other materials available from pharmacists, with details of their manufacturers and suppliers. It is useful for tracking down brand names and the manufacturer who supplies them.

6 When it's not in the library

Interlibrary loans

When you have performed your search you may find that the material you are looking for is not in the library. Most libraries will have access to lists of journals in other libraries or, with the Internet, access to other library OPACs (*see* the section on OPACs in Chapter 2). A library may offer to carry out an interlibrary loan for you. This involves your 'home' library tracking down the material you require and then requesting a loan or copy from the other library. In health libraries this can be carried out at three levels – local, regional and national – and this holds true for other countries as well. A local search involves checking with local libraries for holdings, while a regional search, especially in the NHS, involves checking holdings within an NHS region – most regions will have a regional catalogue of books or serials. On a national level, the library can check holdings within larger libraries, e.g. the British Library DSC, the BMA Library or RSM libraries. This service may be charged for, depending on local policies – copies from all the national libraries have a charge attached and this is reviewed annually.

A similar system operates in the US where the National Network of Libraries of Medicine is co-ordinated by the NLM. This is based on a regional and national network which uses the NLM's DOC-LINE software to request and supply documents. For individual users the interestingly named 'Loansome Doc' provides the same service. Requests can also be routed to international document delivery services such as the Canadian service CISTI (Canada Institute for Scientific and Technical Information) and the British Library DSC.

Document delivery from these providers can now be done not only by post, but also by fax and increasingly by electronic methods to the desktop. Some libraries, especially those in higher education establishments, are using a package called ARIEL, which allows transmission between two computers which have the relevant software. It is worth enquiring with your librarian whether the library has this facility. It should be remembered, however, that the latter methods may cost you more to use as the providers tend to put a premium on this service which is obviously faster than the standard postal response. In future, no doubt, you will be able to get electronic versions of papers delivered direct to your desktop and pay by credit card – indeed the British Library is working towards this system with their *Inside* product (*see* Chapter 4).

Microfilm and microfiche

Many copies, especially of theses and grey literature, can be supplied on microfiche or microfilm. The difference between these formats is fairly straightforward – a microfiche is a single piece of film usually measuring 105 mm by 148 mm on which there can be between 98 and 250 frames, depending on the magnification used. Microfilm is a continuous strip of film, usually 16 mm or 35 mm in width, which can vary in length. It is stored on a spool or cassette in a box.

Although these formats are still considered the best method for preservation of paper materials, it may be difficult to find libraries with the equipment to read them as they are less common than they used to be. Many machines are multipurpose and will handle fiche and film, and many will allow you to make copies on to paper. With microfilm, the spool is usually fed through the light by means of a winding mechanism and the picture projected on to the screen. With fiche, you need to remember that the fiche is put between the two glass sheets (the carrier) with the banner heading towards you. The carrier is then moved to the position where you can see the first page and then across to the required position.

Hints and tips on how to use your librarian

As a practising librarian I felt that it was important to include a section on what a librarian, in an ideal situation, likes to get from a reader by way of an enquiry.

We always want to get as full a reference as possible to materials – and often don't. It is common for readers to turn up wanting an article by Smith that was in the *BMJ* in about 1990 and is possibly about cardiology! It is also not uncommon to eventually discover it was by Jones in the *Lancet* in 1980! References at the end of articles can be wrong so should be treated with care and double-checked for accuracy. An ISSN or ISBN is always useful as that can specify a single book or journal title.

Copying and copyright issues

Questions of copying and copyright occur frequently in any library. Copying is an area that varies between libraries – some libraries still do not charge or only charge a small fee for copying articles or sections from books. In academic libraries or the libraries of most professional societies, a charge is levied based on the cost of materials and wear and tear on the machine. Some larger libraries still offer a service where they will copy articles for you as opposed to self-service, although this is now fairly rare.

Copyright is an emotive issue and is likely to be clouded in the next few years by the European Union legislation. At present the law that applies in the UK is the *Copyright, Designs and Patents Act 1988*. This stipulates the amount that you are allowed to copy from a journal or book. Your library may ask you to sign a copyright declaration form which states that the copy is to be used for the purposes of private study or research and the copy can then be supplied as part of the 'library privilege' scheme. This allows you to take one copy of any one article from one issue of a journal – multiple copies are not allowed unless you pay the copyright clearance fee. Services such as *Inside* from the British Library charge a copyright fee (which can be expensive) and that allows you to copy as many times as you like from one article. From a book, an allowable section is about 1000 words. Your librarian will be able to guide you on this.

Translations

As English is now the international language of medicine, the need for translations of foreign material is not as prevalent as it once was. However, searches on bibliographic databases will throw up the occasional paper which is not in English and which is vital or unique to your research. The British Library has a list of *Journals in Translation* which details those titles which have cover-to-cover translations into English. Many hospitals also keep a list of people willing to undertake translations as part of their programme to provide interpreters for foreign patients. Companies also exist which carry out translations but these can be expensive and unless the paper is vital, should be used with caution.

The Internet

Many users see the Internet as replacing libraries completely. They seem to believe that everything is on the Web, so why should they need to look elsewhere? Although it is true that much information is now on the Internet and that there is probably a website on most subjects, a lot of the information is of dubious quality and some is downright dangerous. A recent goal of health librarians and some healthcare professionals is to try to bring some sort of quality criteria to the Web. Other projects such as *DISCERN* (to be found on website www.discern.org.uk/background.htm) are trying to teach consumers the value of critical appraisal applied to websites. Some of the sites mentioned below are heavily involved in listing quality health sites but as the Web changes from day to day, it would be impossible to list all sites.

Organising Medical Networked Information (OMNI) – www.omni.ac.uk

OMNI was started as one of the e-lib (electronic library) projects by the academic sector funded by the Joint Information Systems Committee (JISC). Its remit was to locate and list quality medical sites on the Internet with an emphasis on UK sites. Over the years it has performed this task using a set of quality criteria and volunteer librarians to locate sites and then write short descriptors of the site plus a link to the site. Currently there are over 4000 resources on *OMNI* which are searchable using a very simple interface or browsable using the NLM classification scheme or a system based on the *UMLS* system (*see* Chapter 2). *OMNI* is now part of the larger *BIOME* (www.biome.ac.uk) project which is looking to provide a gateway to web resources in the life sciences sector.

Medical Matrix – www.medmatrix.org

Medical Matrix was founded by Gary Malet in the US and is a gateway site to medical and health-related resources on the Internet. It contains a very large collection of links to sites of interest and the categories include literature and directories as well as clinical sites.

Health on the Net (HON) – www.hon.ch

Health on the Net is based in Geneva and is designed to realise the benefits of the Internet for healthcare. It contains information of use to the healthcare professional and has a search engine called *MedHunt* which helps track down websites. It indexes sites both manually and automatically and the HON foundation has initiated a code of conduct for health-related websites.

7 The electronic age

Digital libraries

The concept of the 'digital' or 'virtual' library has been around for a couple of years. Depending on who you talk to, the digital library can be a method of electronic access to materials or can include the digitisation of classic works or treasures. As an example of the present thinking on digital libraries I have included the British Library's current approach on the subject.

The British Library is pushing ahead its own digital library plans and among the key corporate goals of the *British Library's Strategic Plan 1999–2002* is that the library will 'place a high priority on collecting digital materials and developing digital library services to ensure our users can consult new forms of publication, and can benefit from the new means of access available through digital and networking technologies'.

The drivers behind this are the development of new electronic forms of publishing and the increasing importance of information and communication technologies. The growing interest in library services for remote users has been fuelled by the rapid expansion of the Internet. The higher education sector is developing access to electronic publications, while publishers, telecommunications companies and information providers have joined forces to explore new opportunities. All these factors are forming a new environment in which libraries will work in the future.

In the *1998 Strategic Review of the British Library*, which led to its new *Strategic Plan*, among the activities to which our users attached highest priority were:

- the inclusion of digital works as an integral part of the collection
- improved access through reading-room services
- improved access through remote document supply services
- improved access through World Wide Web-based services
- preservation and care of the collection in relation to digital materials.

Although these were priorities for the British Library, they form the basis of what libraries mean by the term digital library services.

In addition, digital works are forming an integral part of the British Library's collection. Introduction by the government, when parliamentary time becomes available, of legislation to extend legal deposit will also ensure that the library will begin to develop a national archive of published digital materials. However, until that time, the library has implemented a code of practice for the voluntary deposit of digital works. During this voluntary phase, the library is assessing the burden on publishers of an extension of legal deposit to digital and other non-print forms of publication. It is also developing a digitisation policy to facilitate access to and conservation of collection items.

Therefore the British Library needs to have a digital infrastructure in place in order to satisfy its obligation of maintaining the national published archive, which increasingly will consist of digital publications as well as print publications, and in order to provide ready access to digital materials.

This is by no means only a concern of the British Library. Many university libraries are looking at how they can move into a mixed economy of print and electronic materials, especially with the growth of electronic journals accessed via the Internet.

Electronic journals

Many publishers are making their journals available electronically on the Web. Currently most expect a library to subscribe to both the print and electronic version and this has led to the term 'hybrid library'. Usually a library will subscribe to the print version of a journal and the electronic version is then offered at little or no extra cost. This benefits the user as provision is made for accessing this material away from the library, i.e. at the user's desktop, where the papers can then be printed out. Many people feel that this is the way that print publications will go, with the concept of publishing on demand. Some estimate that in ten years as many as 95% of journals will be made available electronically. Although most of the professional publishing houses are making content available on the Web, this list can only show some of those doing this at present.

British Medical Journal – www.bmj.com

The *BMJ* is somewhat of a rarity in that recent articles are available freely on the Web (the other journal that offers this is the *Journal of Clinical Investigation* through Highwire Press). The electronic version contains most of the material available in the print version but with links to *Medline* and other useful sites.

Health Service Journal – www.hsj.co.uk

The *Health Service Journal* is one of the major journals for healthcare managers. The site on the Web mirrors the weekly published version and has stories, editorials and, of most interest, jobs on-line.

Highwire Press – http://www.highwire.com

Highwire Press was an idea started by Stanford University to publish journals of professional associations on the Web. It began in early 1995 with the on-line production of the weekly *Journal of Biological Chemistry* (*JBC*), the most highly cited (and second largest) peer-reviewed journal. *Science* and *Proceedings of the National Academy of Sciences* soon joined *JBC* on-line. Highwire produces 211 sites on-line, with many more planned. The site includes journals that you have to pay for in order to access current content but many have a policy of offering older material free.

Elsevier *Science Direct* – http://www.sciencedirect.com/

As a major publisher in science, technology and medicine, Elsevier is putting much of its journal material up on the Web for libraries and subscribers. The *Science Direct* website covers some 1100 journals in 16 subject areas. The service also allows users to link between references in articles on *Science Direct* with other cited publications in full text. Articles can be downloaded and printed in PDF format.

PubMed Central – http://www.pubmedcentral.nih.gov/

A new project was proposed in 1999 called *PubMed Central*, in which articles would be published on the Web in the same way that nuclear physics articles have been published via the Los Alamos site for some years now. This concept was also mirrored in the biosciences in Europe by *E-Biosci* led by the European Molecular Biology Organization (EMBO – www.embo.org). The original idea has been slightly changed in the light of feedback from publishers and the thorny problem of peer review in a web environment. *PubMed Central* now looks to be a repository of electronic materials which have been deposited by publishers after six months or longer. Currently five journals have signed up to deposit their text and another seven are in the pipeline, including the *BMJ*.

The other big question at present occupying libraries and librarians is how should electronic materials such as journals be archived for posterity and who should do it? Is this the job of the library or the publisher? And how do you keep a record of websites at any particular moment in time which may be of use in medico-legal cases? Two projects looking at this problem are *JSTOR* in the US and *NESLI* in the UK. Many libraries and librarians are looking to these two projects and to the national libraries for some sort of guidance.

Multimedia

A huge amount of health-related material is now available as 'multimedia' on CD-ROM and the Web. Multimedia refers to the fact that the product will contain a number of different media such as text, sound, images and video clips. Many of the products offered are far from 'multi' media, being perhaps a textbook put on to CD-ROM with pictures and diagrams – some also claim to be interactive but are far from it. Most are concerned with anatomical and physiological topics as these lend themselves very well to multimedia presentation. Increasingly, libraries are offering multimedia products to users, a good example being the Royal College of Surgeons, which has a collection of multimedia training products and a special area put aside for people to consult them. It would be unhelpful to list all those available, but some of the better ones are described below.

Animated Dissection of Anatomy in Medicine (ADAM)

ADAM Interactive Anatomy is an interactive learning and teaching CD-ROM based on anatomical illustrations of the complete human body, which enhances the study of human anatomy and related topics. This is the 'flagship' product in the ADAM Scholar Series, which is the successor to both ADAM Comprehensive and ADAM Standard. It provides many new enhancements derived from extensive input from teachers, authors, health professionals and students. The product has been spun off into a number of smaller products that focus on particular areas of the body or particular processes, such as pregnancy. The results are very impressive and it is a truly interactive product which you will find in some of the major teaching hospitals.

Interactive Skeleton

This program from Primal Pictures features a dynamic 3-D skeleton model which is presented in the most outstanding and realistic topographical detail. Users navigate their way round the model in all directions or focus on specific areas and bones as they choose. Users can work with the complete skeleton or take it apart and home in on certain bones or sections. All areas of muscle and tendon are shown and there is comprehensive labelling of structures. It also includes comprehensive indices and a file-linking system with a self-test programme. Interactive Skeleton won the BMA Award for Best Electronic Product.

Wellcome Series on Tropical Medicine

The Wellcome Trust has produced a series of interactive CD-ROMs on various tropical diseases aimed at students in developed and developing countries. These disks are relatively inexpensive and are very comprehensive. They cover subjects such as leprosy, malaria and trypanosomiasis.

AV materials

Film and video have also been popular for some time in healthcare education. A few years ago Graves Medical Audio-visual Service provided a comprehensive loans service for AV materials but they ceased to trade and so getting this type of material became a lot harder. Many libraries carry a selection of materials they have obtained and these may include the old-fashioned tape slide materials that were popular in the early 1980s. The BMA Library took up the challenge of providing a major collection of AV materials and it now provides a loan service for videos of health topics. It also tapes relevant television programmes and runs an awards scheme for outstanding films and videos on health topics. It publishes a catalogue of its holdings, copies of which are available from the library. It would be the first point of enquiry when looking for video and film material.

The Wellcome Trust also has a photographic library and a huge collection of photographic materials, both modern and historic. It will also undertake photography from the materials housed in the Wellcome Institute for the History of Medicine's collections.

The *British National Film and Video Guide* (*BNFVG*) is a full listing by subject of films and videos available for non-theatrical loan or purchase, together with distributor address information as supplied by the National Film and Television Archive of the British Film Institute. The guide includes details of over 500 films and videos, including documentaries, feature films, educational and training films, and television programmes. *BNFVG* is available on annual subscription. Issues are published quarterly, cumulating in an annual volume which includes records and indexes for the whole year. Each subscription also comes with a printed index to the Universal Decimal Classification subject headings used in the guide.

8 How to appraise your findings

How to appraise a paper

Much work has been done as part of the 'evidence-based' movement on critical appraisal skills for both healthcare professionals and librarians. What is critical appraisal and what is the difference between 'critically appraising' an article and simply reading it? If you have done a literature search and copied an article, why can't you just read it rather than doing a critical appraisal ?

Critical appraisal is basically a technique that offers a way of increasing the effectiveness of your reading by enabling you to quickly reject papers that are of too poor a quality to inform practice and systematically to evaluate those that you accept so that you can extract their useful points.

Critical appraisal can provide solutions to three of the major problems in health information:

- information overload: the sheer volume of material now being published
- the '80/20 rule': the fact that much material is of limited relevance and use in providing clinical care and so the information you need resides in only a small fraction of this huge mass
- nihilism: the problem that all studies are flawed to some extent, or are too 'ivory tower' to make much difference to 'real life'

Although it depends to a certain extent on what sort of article you are appraising, there are always three basic stages:

- the message: what are the findings of this article?
- the validity: are the conclusions justified by the description of the methodology and the findings?
- the utility: can I generalise the findings to my patients? Are my patients sufficiently like those in the study to extrapolate the findings?

Utility is in some ways the hardest to be rigidly scientific about and making decisions here may still be an art. For instance, although the paper is scientifically faultless, you may be left pondering several questions.

- If the selection criteria included 'age 70–80', can I use the conclusions for patients in the 65–70 age groups, and what about the relatively fit and 'biologically young' 81-year-olds?
- Can studies on urban Americans be extrapolated from say New York to York, and are rural practices in Scandinavia different to those in Scotland?

Appraisal of original research

This approach applies to primary studies of original research. You start by skimming through to get the flavour of the article and then analyse it more slowly, beginning with three screening questions to see if it passes your criteria for closer scrutiny. Also, it is useful to find out if the journal is peer-reviewed, although this process is now under question especially with the rise of e-servers (*PubMed Central*). It is usually stated in the instructions to authors if the journal is peer-reviewed and this should suggest quality, but it is no absolute guarantee of scientific rigour. If the authors have included a literature review to put the study in context, is the review current, comprehensive and balanced?

1 The message

- What is the message to take back to clinical practice? What is the bottom line?

2 The validity

Start with three basic screening questions.

- Did the trial address a clearly focused issue?
- How was the sample selected? Is it big enough, and is it representative? Was it a randomised controlled trial (the gold standard)?
- Were all the patients who entered the trial properly accounted for at its conclusion? Were any who swapped groups analysed using 'intention to treat'?

If you get a *yes* to all three, then continue to ascertain the meaning of the article by looking for further answers.

- Are there any differences between the two groups in terms of selection bias or variables which could explain the differences between them (factors like age, sex and social class)?

- Blinding: Were the patients, workers or study personnel 'blind to the treatment'? Beware of potential breaches of blinding (e.g. perhaps a taste difference between drug and placebo).
- Were the groups similar at the start of the trial (in terms of age, sex and any variables, such as smoking rates in a cardiovascular diseases study)?
- Apart from the experimental intervention, were the groups treated equally?

Finally you should consider the results.

- How large was the treatment effect (consider what outcomes were recorded and how the differences between the groups were expressed)?
- How precise was the estimate of the treatment effects (i.e. look for confidence intervals)?

You should look out for very obscure statistical tests or the use of parametric tests where the data do not justify them. Beware of 'statistically significant' results which are not 'clinically significant'.

3 The utility

- Can the results be applied to the local population? How different are the patients in the study population from yours?
- Were all the clinically important outcomes considered? If any were neglected, does this affect the interpretation?
- Are the benefits worth the harms and costs? This is a bit of an 'extra'; much research will not include cost benefit analyses, but may be useful if you are looking at different management options.

Appraisal of reviews

This format is useful for the secondary literature that synthesises or integrates information from multiple primary literature sources. These can be meta-analyses, reviews, overviews, systematic reviews, guidelines or economic analyses. Unfortunately, these techniques cannot overcome the problem of publication bias. Papers with positive conclusions are more likely to be published than ones with negative conclusions. Positive studies may also produce duplicate publications, with no clear acknowledgement that they are analysing the same group of patients. However, when people produce a meta-analysis of all studies on a particular topic, because the 'grey literature' can be harder to find, the meta-analysis may be over-optimistic about new therapies.

It is useful to remember that a systematic review is an overview of primary research studies that reach specific standards in terms of methodology. It should be explicit about **how** the reviewers located the studies and which **exclusion** and **inclusion** criteria they used. A meta-analysis is a mathematical synthesis of the results of two or more primary studies that addressed the same research question and used comparable methodologies.

1 The message

- Does the review set out to answer a precise question about patient care?

2 The validity

Have the authors looked for studies using:

- *Medline* and other relevant bibliographic databases
- Cochrane controlled clinical trials register
- foreign-language literature
- 'grey literature'
- citation searching using any articles found
- personal approaches to experts in the field to find unpublished reports
- hand searches of the relevant specialised journals?

For meta-analysis it may be important to track down the raw study data for re-analysis.

Also, have the authors included explicit inclusion and exclusion criteria for studies, taking account of the patients in the studies, the interventions used, the outcomes recorded and the methodology?

In a meta-analysis how are the results presented? In practice, the results are often displayed graphically as horizontal lines representing the 95% confidence intervals of the effect of each trial. Sometimes there is a 'blob' in the middle representing the single best estimate of the intervention found by that study (the blobbogram). The results of the meta-analysis are represented by a diamond. These are sometimes called forest plots.

Have the authors considered the idea that the studies are sufficiently similar in their design, interventions and subjects to merit combination?

3 The utility

This may be easier than for a piece of original research. The various studies may have used patients of different ages or social classes, but if the treatment effects are consistent across the studies, then generalisation to other groups or populations is more justified.

However, be wary of subgroup analyses where the authors attempt to draw new conclusions by comparing the outcomes for patients in one study with the patients in another study, rather than trying to draw together the patients in the control and intervention groups in each study. Such conclusions have often later been shown to be artefacts and not justified. Also, be wary of 'data-dredging' exercises, testing multiple hypotheses against the data, especially if the hypotheses were constructed after the study had begun data collection.

You may also want to ask more questions.

- Were all clinically important outcomes considered?
- Are the benefits worth the harms and costs?

Collections of appraised articles

For some articles you may be lucky enough to find a 'model answer' in the form of an expert commentary or a published critical appraisal. Any of these are traceable through the excellent *Netting the Evidence* website at http://www.shef.ac.uk/~scharr/ir/netting/.

Critical appraisal is a mixture of the **science** of examining validity and the **art** of assessing utility. There are a number of unresolved questions you might like to think about.

- Declaration of outside interests or commercial sponsorship: how would you regard the report of a project funded by a pharmaceutical company who marketed some of the drugs involved?
- Would you use the results of studies which were methodologically sound but where you felt there were ethical problems and no explicit evidence of Ethics Committee approval?

- How 'applicable' are the results of meta-analyses to the care of individual patients?
- How do you 'square the circle' when a meta-analysis and a randomised controlled trial in the same area produce conflicting results, or worse still two meta-analyses disagree?

Training

Training has been available for some time on critical appraisal skills. Some of the courses offered are listed below.

- There are an increasing number of locally available critical appraisal workshops, for instance in Trent Region you can contact: The School of Health and Related Research (ScHARR), Sheffield University, 30 Regent Court, Sheffield S1 1DA; tel: 0114 222 0797, fax: 0114 272 4095.
- The Critical Appraisal Skills Programme from the Public Health Resources Unit at Oxford.
- There is a module at the University of Leeds which has been designed to provide a basic introduction to the systematic literature review process. It follows the NHS Centre for Reviews and Dissemination Guidelines for systematic reviews and includes a self-assessment questionnaire for evaluating learning outcomes.

The users' guides to the medical literature

A very good set of guides to using the literature was published in the *Journal of the American Medical Association* (*JAMA*), beginning in 1993. Some are now available on the Web with clinical scenarios and worked examples of question answering at http://www.cche.net/principles/content_all.asp

Each includes a checklist of questions to use in critical appraisal and some also include advice about the best *Medline* search strategy. For some of these topics expert search strategies are available from the Oxford Institute of Health Studies Library, which will help you optimise retrieval of documents from databases such as *Medline*. There are also filters on *PubMed* (*see above*) to help with retrieving the most useful information and most health libraries can help with setting up search strategies to optimise your retrieval of relevant materials.

Quality and the Internet

This is currently a huge area of concern with spurious information appearing on the Internet as well as useful information about rare conditions. The ease of self-publishing and the lack of peer review has led to a proliferation of medical information on the Internet to the extent that health is the second most popular topic on the Web (after sex!). Problems include: the indiscriminate, unwieldy retrieval of material from search engines, which mostly lacks context; the prevalence of word 'spamming' or 'spamdexing' through the repetition of keywords; and inclusion of spurious keywords. This has serious implications for relevancy ranking with search engines.

The *BMJ* of 17 August 1996 (**313** (7054): 381) published an article by Hilary Bower which found that the Internet was seeing the growth of unverified health claims such as the sites that claimed that shark cartilage inhibits tumour growth and cancer, and that melatonin claimed to strengthen the body's immune system. The American College of Gastroenterology concluded that 'Surfing the Net May be Hazardous to Your Health'.

The reliability of health information is also of concern. The *BMJ* paper of 28 June 1997 (**314**: 1875) by Impicciatore *et al.* 'The reliability of health information for the public on the world wide web: systematic survey of advice on managing fever in children at home' concluded that 'only a few web sites provided complete and accurate information for this common and widely discussed condition. This suggests an urgent need to check public oriented healthcare information on the internet for accuracy, completeness, and consistency'.

The difficulties with evaluating web pages can be summarised as:

- they cannot be browsed in the same way as print
- they tend not to have a set of common features (such as statement of responsibility, introduction, preface, table of contents, index)
- there are time and cost implications with Web access.

However, a lot of work is currently being done on quality evaluation of Internet sites. Several of the sites mentioned elsewhere in this book have already put together quality criteria by which sites are judged before being included on their gateways. Two of the most useful sites are *OMNI* (http://www.omni.ac.uk) and *Health on the*

Net (http://www.hon.ch/). These publish their criteria for inclusion and *Health on the Net* awards a kitemark for sites that agree to meet their quality criteria. The European Union-funded project Towards European Accreditation and Certification of Health Telematics Services (TEAC-Health) included Internet sites as one of its three areas of research and study. Its literature reviews, working papers and final conclusions can be found at www.multimedica.com/TEAC.

Also of interest are a number of reviews.

- The *BMJ* has published criteria for evaluating health-related websites which are available at http://www.bmj.com/cgi/content/full/318/7184/647#.
- *DISCERN*, which is an instrument for judging the quality of written consumer health information on treatment choices, can be found at http://www.discern.org.uk/. This is a checklist of 16 questions for consumers and patients to evaluate websites, developed, standardised and validated by working with 13 national self-help groups; however, it can be very time-consuming and subjective. Also, it seems to assume that consumers accept that care should be based on objective studies and understand principles of 'evidence-based practice'.
- MedCertain is another quality rating system using 'MedPICS', which is a system for certification and rating of trustworthy and assessed health information on the Net.

Certain criteria can be used when assessing websites.

1 The context of the website

- Audience – who are the audience for the information on the website, patients or healthcare professionals?
- Authority – look at the URL for the site: '.com' and '.co' addresses suggest commercial bodies; '.org' suggests non-profit-making sites; '.edu' and '.ac' suggest academic institutions; '.gov', '.doh', etc. suggest government departments. A '~name' in the URL may indicate a personal home page. It is useful to 'skip back' through the URL to parent pages to find if the parent body is trustworthy.
- Provenance – what is the history of the site? Who has owned it?

2 The content of the website

- Coverage – how comprehensive is the coverage of the topic?
- Accuracy – how accurate is the information contained on the website?
- Uniqueness – is the information unique in any way?
- Currency/update frequency and regularity – an important concern and a useful tool for judging the value of a site. With the average lifespan of a website being only 75 days, it is important that the information is kept up to date.

3 Access to the website

- Accessibility – are there any access restrictions to the site or is there a need for special requirements such as Internet Explorer 5.0?
- Use of graphics – is there excessive use of graphics and sound? This slows down the retrieval time for a site and may put off potential users.
- Design and layout/user interface – is this good and easy to read? The Bobby scores indicate how user-friendly a site is for visually impaired readers.
- User support/documentation – how good is this?

Triangulation

Triangulation is a research technique which can be applied to the critical appraisal of literature. A study may employ more than one sampling strategy and also more than one type of data. Triangulation is a term taken from land surveying – if you know a single landmark you may know where you are along a line, but if you know two landmarks then you can locate yourself more accurately at the intersection of these two lines.

There are four basic types of triangulation:

1. data triangulation – the use of a variety of data sources in a study
2. investigator triangulation – the use of several different researchers or evaluators
3. theory triangulation – the use of multiple perspectives to interpret a single set of data

4 methodological triangulation – the use of multiple methods to study a single problem.

Triangulation is obviously ideal but can be expensive and time-consuming. One important strategy for conducting evaluation research is to use multiple methods, measurements and perspectives from a variety of researchers where practically possible. In the social sciences much research depends on a combination of observations, interviewing and literature analysis. Studies that rely on only one method are more vulnerable to errors linked to that particular methodology than studies that use multiple methods, in which different data types provide a method of cross-checking validity. Triangulation can include borrowing and combining parts from pure methodological approaches, thus creating mixed methodological strategies; any given study could include several measurement approaches, varying design approaches and varying analytical approaches to achieve triangulation.

Therefore we can see that critical appraisal of the literature found in the health library can lead to a more analytical way of using the material retrieved from a search.

Further reading

Crombie IM (1996) *The Pocket Guide to Critical Appraisal.* BMJ Publishing Group, London.

Greenhalgh T (1997) *How to Read a Paper: the basis of evidence-based medicine.* BMJ Publishing Group, London.

Jones R and Kinmouth AL (1995) *Critical Reading for Primary Care.* Oxford University Press, Oxford.

Ong BN (1996) *Rapid Appraisal and Health Policy.* Chapman and Hall, London.

Roberts R (1999) *Information for Evidence-based Care. Harnessing Health Care Information Series No. 1.* Radcliffe Medical Press, Oxford.

9 The future

Introduction

What will happen to the concept of the library during this century? Will books disappear, apart from those that are seen as 'treasures' and put into museum settings? Will the library be seen as the museum of the book? Will a library be just a collection of computer terminals? Or will they just disappear altogether? With the appearance of the electronic book or e-book, will readers be able to download all of their key texts for study from the Internet and never have to visit a library unless they are doing historical research? Or will readers just have their key facts on an e-book and still consult journals and other materials in the library? One project – *Project Gutenberg* – is aiming to put all of the classic literature on to the Web for downloading on to a laptop computer for reading purposes.

These topics are currently exercising librarians in all fields and I can only give some idea of the way libraries may evolve in the future as a support to learning. Many librarians may disagree with my analysis but I believe the following major themes will affect libraries in the future.

Consumer health information and informatics

Consumer health information is not a new concept, it has been around in some form since the 1970s when most of the original work was done. However, in the UK, it took on a new lease of life when the *Patient's Charter* was released by the government in the early 1990s. This gave more emphasis to patient empowerment and the concept that the patient needed access to information about the best possible treatment. This has also been taken up by the 'evidence-based' movement and there is now a stipulation that the information should be based on the best possible evidence. One of the leading UK lights in the consumer health movement is the Help for Health Trust which now runs the Centre for Health Information Quality and looks at the quality of information given to patients as leaflets and whether it is evidence-based or not.

From the consumer health movement developed the concept of

Health Information Services which were based in NHS regions in the mid-1990s. These gave basic information to patients about their diagnosis and treatment. In the late 1990s these services evolved into NHS Direct, the nurse-based telephone triage system and *NHS Direct Online*, the web-based service (http://www.nhsdirect.nhs.uk/).

Information technology is playing a more important role in consumer health information with the appearance of touch-screen systems based in hospitals and planned for supermarkets and stations, an example being Start Here, which has been trialled at the Whittington Hospital in London. In the US there is increasingly more interest in getting information to patients through services such as *PubMed* and *Medline Plus*, both from the NLM (http://www.nlm.nih.gov). *Healthfinder* (http://www.healthfinder.gov/) is an excellent US government website which provides consumer health information.

The role of the library in these situations is probably to provide access to the most relevant sites and to help provide more in-depth articles when required. The medical profession is also beginning to encounter patients who are now better informed about their own conditions and are demanding different treatments and the ability to contact the doctor electronically.

Health informatics

Informatics is the study of information technology and health informatics is the application of this technology to health. Increasingly, health informatics and health librarianship are moving closer together as projects such as the Integrated Academic Information Management System (IAIMS) aim to put information resources, such as *Medline*, on the doctor's desktop computer linked to the patient record. This appears to be the case in the US where the NLM funds much of the informatics research, but in the UK we have been less keen to work with our IT colleagues, although this is now changing, especially with the publication of the strategy document *Information for Health*.

The role of the library in the move towards health informatics is to look at applying library skills to information retrieval problems and linking bibliographical systems with data systems. There is also still a need for education and training even when the information is brought to the health professional's desktop.

National Electronic Library for Health (NeLH) – http://www.nelh.nhs.uk

The NeLH was also proposed in the *Information for Health* strategy document. The idea is based on the metaphor of a library on four floors: the Knowledge Floor, the Know-How Floor, the Patients' Floor (currently *NHS Direct Online*) and the Knowledge Management Floor. The Knowledge Floor will contain access to databases and published materials, the Know-How Floor will look at guidelines and the Knowledge Management Floor will deal with training and education issues and how to perform searches, etc. An atrium is also part of the 'library' and will be an area with a help desk and a place that professionals can meet to discuss problems. Virtual branch libraries are also being built in specific areas such as cancer and heart disease.

A Librarian Development Programme is running alongside the NeLH to educate librarians better in helping to deliver the NeLH.

Clinical librarianship

The concept of clinical librarianship is not a new one. Two projects were originally carried out at Guy's Hospital in London in the early 1980s to look at the idea of librarians being part of the clinical team and delivering information to the bedside to aid in patient treatment. At the time it was felt to be a success but the idea did not take off in the UK, unlike the US, where clinical librarianship programmes are common. It may have been that the technology at the time (dumb terminals and postal request systems) meant that the librarian had to return to the library to perform the search and get the printouts. However, the US experience and the fact that City Hospital in Nottingham has been running a service for a number of years, plus a recent experiment at the John Radcliffe Hospital in Oxford with the 'evidence cart', have proven that the system does work and technology now makes it possible to deliver clinical librarian services to the team at the bedside.

Telemedicine

The delivery of diagnosis remotely using telemedicine may also impinge on how information is delivered to both patients and the health professional involved in a consultation. It is an area where librarians should work with their technical colleagues to see how relevant information can be delivered alongside medical images to the patient and the consulting doctor. Some examples of useful and innovative sites are the *Telemedicine Information Exchange* in the US (http://tie.telemed.org/) and the *UK National Database of Telemedicine* at the University of Portsmouth (http://www.dis.port.ac.uk/ndtm/).

Virtual reality

Virtual reality (VR) may belong firmly in the world of computer graphics and visualisation, but it is being used in the world of medicine and library guiding. The British Library developed a programme in the early 1990s to show people around the new St Pancras building but never developed it beyond concept stage. VR has been suggested for training surgeons in techniques without injuring real patients and for delivering telemedicine. The delivery of information and different ways of visualising information may well belong in the fields of VR; projects such as the Visible Human Project developed by the NLM (http://www.nlm.nih.gov) where a male and female cadaver have been scanned using magnetic resonance imaging (MRI) and computerised tomography (CT) and then microtomed, may give enough data to create virtual medical environments to develop new techniques in microsurgery and even nanosurgery. Another project which has been developed is the idea of an 'Information Wall' where concepts are placed like bricks in a virtual wall and you can rearrange the bricks and move the wall about to combine retrieval techniques.

Interactive television

Many people see consumer health information as deliverable on interactive television. Several television companies are now developing medical channels to deliver educational materials to healthcare professionals, and satellite systems are certainly being used to deliver health training and to look into the possibility of delivering information to developing countries. One such company is Medical Network News which has installations in developed countries but is looking to deliver its product to developing countries. The bandwidth it uses is such that speedy delivery of electronic full text is a distinct possibility – will librarians abandon their photocopiers and replace them with scanners?

Conclusions

Obviously this can only be one particular viewpoint, and a technically minded one at that, of the future for libraries. Many of these concepts are already happening. The move to electronic materials has already started, although many readers still prefer print to electronic means – after all, as one recent respondent in a questionnaire from the British Library said, 'you can't take a laptop into the bath with you'!

Index